Fast Facts

Fast Facts:
Rhinitis

Second edition

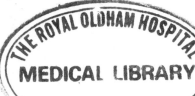

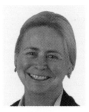

Glenis K Scadding MA MD FRCP
Royal National Throat, Nose and Ear Hospital
London, UK

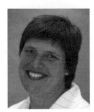

Wytske J Fokkens MD PhD
Department of Otorhinolaryngology
Academic Medical Centre, University of Amsterdam
Amsterdam, The Netherlands

Declaration of Independence
This book is as balanced and as practical as we can make it.
Ideas for improvement are always welcome: feedback@fastfacts.com

An independent publication
provided as a service to medicine by

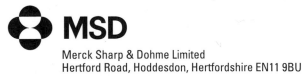

MSD

Merck Sharp & Dohme Limited
Hertford Road, Hoddesdon, Hertfordshire EN11 9BU

11-11 SGA.09.GB.13589.O

HEALTH PRESS

Fast Facts: Rhinitis
First published (as Fast Facts: Allergic Rhinitis) 2000
Second edition 2007
Reprinted 2008, December 2009

Health Press Limited, Elizabeth House, Queen Street, Abingdon,
Oxford OX14 3LN, UK
Tel: +44 (0)1235 523233
Fax: +44 (0)1235 523238

Book orders can be placed by telephone or via the website.
For regional distributors or to order via the website, please go to:
www.fastfacts.com
For telephone orders, please call +44 (0)1752 202301 (UK and Europe),
1 800 247 6553 (USA, toll free), +1 419 281 1802 (Americas) or +61 (0)2 9351 6173
(Asia–Pacific).

Fast Facts is a trademark of Health Press Limited.

The publisher and the authors have made every effort to ensure the accuracy of this
book, but cannot accept responsibility for any errors or omissions.

For all drugs, please consult the product labeling approved in your country for
prescribing information.

A CIP record for this title is available from the British Library.

ISBN 978-1-905832-06-4

Author: Scadding, GK (Glenis)
Fast Facts: Rhinitis/
Glenis K Scadding, Wytske J Fokkens

The cover shows a false-color scanning electron micrograph of a pollen grain of the
garden hollyhock, *Althaea rosa*. Dr Jeremy Burgess/Science Photo Library

Medical illustrations by Dee McLean, London, UK,
and Annamaria Dutto, Withernsea, UK.
Typesetting and page layout by Zed, Oxford, UK.
Printed by Latimer Trend & Company Limited, Plymouth, UK.

FSC

Mixed Sources
Product group from well-managed
forests and other controlled sources

Cert no. SGS-COC-005493
www.fsc.org
© 1996 Forest Stewardship Council

Text printed on biodegradable and recyclable paper manufactured
using elemental chlorine free (ECF) wood pulp from well-managed
forests.

Glossary of abbreviations

ACE inhibitor: angiotensin-converting enzyme inhibitor

ARIA: Allergic Rhinitis and its Impact on Asthma (an initiative of the World Health Organization and other groups)

ASA: acetylsalicylic acid (aspirin)

AU: allergy units

BU: biological units

EAACI: European Academy of Allergology and Clinical Immunology

eNO: exhaled nitric oxide

ENT: ear, nose and throat

FEV$_1$: forced expiratory volume in 1 minute

GM-CSF: granulocyte-macrophage colony-stimulating factor

ICAM: intercellular adhesion molecule

Ig: immunoglobulin

IL: interleukin

NARES: non-allergic rhinitis with eosinophilia

nNO: nasal nitric oxide

NO: nitric oxide

NSAID: non-steroidal anti-inflammatory drug

OME: otitis media with effusion

PCD: primary ciliary dyskinesia

RAST: radioallergosorbent test

SPT: skin-prick test

Th$_1$: T helper 1 (cells)

Th$_2$: T helper 2 (cells)

WHO: World Health Organization

Introduction

Allergic diseases have been described as a modern epidemic, with over 20% of the total population suffering from allergic rhinitis, asthma or atopic eczema. Of these diseases, allergic rhinitis is the most common and the most underdiagnosed and mistreated.

The effects of the symptoms of rhinitis, allergic or otherwise, on quality of life, particularly through sleep disturbance, are beginning to be appreciated. The long-term effects of poor school and examination performance are beginning to be investigated. The comorbidity of allergic rhinitis with asthma – the 'one airway' hypothesis – is generally accepted, but other relevant comorbidities involving the eyes, throat, ears and voice are still being elucidated. Studies suggest that accurate diagnosis of rhinitis and effective treatment can reduce other chest and ear, nose and throat problems.

Severely affected individuals are treated by specialists in allergy, lung medicine, pediatrics, otorhinolaryngology and dermatology. The majority of people, however, are seen by generalists or by specialists in other fields. We have written this short and practically oriented text on rhinitis, including not only allergic but other forms of rhinitis plus acute and chronic rhinosinusitis, nasal polyposis and comorbidities such as asthma, adenoid hypertrophy and otitis media with effusion, for these practitioners. We hope that it will enable them to optimize their treatment and to know when and to whom to refer those with difficult disease.

1 Allergy: an increasing problem

Allergy is common: 20–40% of the population of the industrialized world have a positive skin-prick test for allergens, and 15–20% will develop an atopic disease (see below). The prevalence of atopic diseases is highest among teenagers.

Allergy is common in very young children, though it can be difficult to discriminate it from recurrent viral upper airway disease. In Germany, 6% of children under 2 years old were found to be sensitized to grass and 3% were sensitized to house dust mite; in 40% of children, allergic rhinitis started before the age of 6 years, and 80% developed symptoms before the age of 20.

The risk of developing allergic disease is influenced by genetic and environmental factors (Figure 1.1).

Genetic factors

'Atopy' refers to a genetic predisposition to produce immunoglobulin E (IgE) in response to minute amounts of environmental protein allergens. Non-atopic individuals can produce IgE, but normally do so only transiently. In atopic individuals, the production continues and leads to various atopic disorders, such as:

- atopic dermatitis or eczema
- asthma
- allergic rhinitis.

A highly atopic person is affected early in life, developing atopic dermatitis soon after birth; asthma and allergic rhinitis develop subsequently. This is sometimes called the 'atopic march'.

On the other hand, a person who becomes allergic to pollen in adolescence has a low degree of atopy and is less likely to be troubled by eczema. However, progression from seasonal rhinitis to a more persistent form and to rhinosinusitis and asthma is now increasingly recognized.

With one atopic parent, the risk of atopy in the child is doubled, with maternal influence being greater than paternal. If both parents are

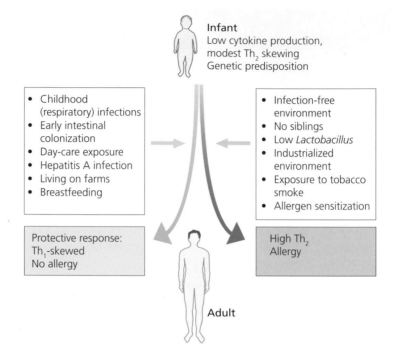

Figure 1.1 Different factors influence the development of allergic disease. Early childhood contact with infectious agents may protect against allergies. Thus, factors that increase the likelihood of this (e.g. day-care exposure, a less hygienic living environment – as indicated by hepatitis A infection) are associated with protection, while factors that decrease the likelihood of early infection (e.g. being a first-born or an only child) are associated with an increased risk of developing allergy. Th_1/Th_2, T helper 1/2 (cells).

atopic, the risk is quadrupled. Several genes are involved and children probably inherit predispositions: for atopic disease in general, for specific organ involvement and for disease severity. Thus, a child with one parent with hay fever is likely to be less severely affected than one whose parents have severe eczema and asthma.

Environmental exposure
A low concordance rate for atopy among monozygotic twins shows that genetic inheritance is not the sole arbiter of the atopic state. Birth immediately before a pollen season leads to a slightly increased risk of

pollen allergy. This is probably because allergen exposure occurs at a time when the immune system is immature and vulnerable.

Allergic rhinitis, atopic dermatitis and asthma have increased in prevalence in Western and westernized countries in the past 30–40 years (Figures 1.2 and 1.3). The reasons are unknown, but suggestions include:
- a decrease in the rate of infection
- an increase in exposure to allergens, pollution and irritants (e.g. smoke, gas)
- changes in diet, with a reduction in the intake of protective nutrients
- an increase in stress.

Decreases in infection. The hygiene hypothesis proposes that insufficient stimulation of the immune system by early childhood infections leads to an enhanced risk of developing allergic disease. A switch from protective, IgG-type immune reactions (mediated by T helper 1 cells; Th_1) to allergic, IgE-type reactions (involving T helper 2 cells; Th_2) in response to decreased infection in early years has been postulated.

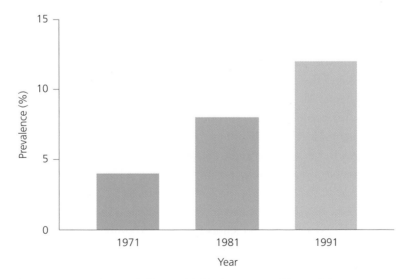

Figure 1.2 Prevalence of allergic rhinitis in 18-year-old Swedish men. Reproduced with permission from Åberg N. Asthma and allergic rhinitis in Swedish conscripts. *Clin Exp Allergy* 1989;19:59–63.

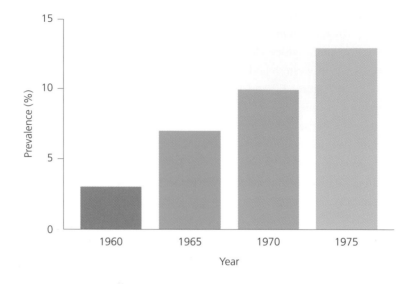

Figure 1.3 Prevalence of eczema in young Danish school children. Reproduced with permission from Schultz Larsen F, Hanifin JM. Secular change in the occurrence of atopic dermatitis. *Acta Derm Venereol Suppl* (Stockh) 1992;176:7–12.

T helper cell subsets are characterized by their cytokine profile: Th_1 synthesize interleukin-2 (IL-2) and interferon-γ, while Th_2 produce IL-3, IL-4, IL-5 and IL-13 (see Figure 3.3, page 25).

The Th_1 and Th_2 systems were thought to be mutually suppressive. In fact, it has been recognized that both Th_1-mediated (autoimmune) disorders and Th_2-mediated (allergic) disorders have increased in prevalence over the past decades. The problem is now thought to be one of immune dysregulation, possibly relating to a failure of suppression of T cell responses by T regulatory cells.

One of the fundamental tenets of this hypothesis is that changes in lifestyle have contributed to a reduction in the exposure of individual children to microorganisms. Seasonal allergic rhinitis is more common in first-born children and in those born into higher social classes – groups less likely to be in contact with infected people. Seasonal allergic rhinitis is also less common in those with hepatitis A antibody, which is a marker for unhygienic living.

Patterns of gut bacteria may also be relevant. The use of antibiotics in early life increases the relative risk of being atopic. Gut flora differs between Estonia, where atopy is rare, and Sweden, where it is common. The use of probiotics such as *Lactobacillus* is under investigation as a means of reducing immune dysregulation.

Allergen exposure. There is convincing evidence that the prevalence of atopic disease increases when people move to westernized countries from native environments. This could relate to increased exposure to house dust mites in carpeted, centrally heated and poorly ventilated homes or to changes in diet or incidence of infections. Exposure to grass pollen has fallen with increased silage production, yet concomitantly the incidence of hay fever has risen, suggesting that high allergen levels are not causative. Indeed, there is now known to be a bell-shaped curve for sensitization in relation to allergen exposure, with maximal sensitization at moderate allergen levels and tolerance at very high and very low doses.

Pollution exposure. Both indoor pollution (parental smoking, gas heating) and outdoor pollution (diesel exhaust particles, nitrogen dioxide) can provoke wheezing in sensitized individuals. The role of pollution in allergic sensitization remains in dispute. Recent studies suggest that the combination of air pollution and sunlight may be important in the development of asthma. Laboratory experiments suggest that pollutants such as nitrogen dioxide and ozone increase the inflammatory response caused by allergen exposure. However, atopic diseases were more common in affluent Munich (former West Germany) than in Leipzig (former East Germany), despite the greater industrial pollution (coal gas, sulfur dioxide) in the latter, so the type of pollutant appears to be relevant.

Dietary changes. The role of diet has proved difficult to elucidate, but there is some evidence for a reduction in inflammation with a diet rich in omega-3 fatty acids and, possibly, for decreased allergic disease with an antioxidant-rich diet.

Timing of dietary exposure may be crucial. Avoiding peanuts during pregnancy and while breastfeeding has not decreased the incidence of peanut allergy in children, and nor has avoiding peanuts during early childhood. Research in this area continues: for example, a randomized study is comparing the rate of sensitization in susceptible children exposed to oral peanut as young babies with the rate in those not exposed.

The route of exposure to food allergens may also be relevant in determining the nature of the immunologic response – there is some evidence that peanut sensitization occurs via the skin, particularly the broken epidermis of eczematous areas if treated with creams or ointments containing arachis (peanut) oil.

Stress is popularly thought to increase allergic sensitization and/or clinical expression. Evidence is beginning to appear for psychoneuroimmunologic connections.

Allergic rhinitis

Allergic rhinitis is a global health problem, affecting 10 to 25% of the population. This figure probably underestimates the prevalence of the disease, as many individuals do not recognize rhinitis as a disease and do not consult a physician.

Allergic rhinitis has been identified as one of the top ten reasons for visits to primary care clinics. Although it is not usually a severe disease, it alters significantly the social life of individuals and affects school performance and work productivity. Moreover, the costs incurred as a result of rhinitis are substantial. The possible association between allergic rhinitis and other conditions including asthma, sinusitis, otitis media, nasal polyposis, lower respiratory tract infection and even dental malocclusion should be considered in evaluating the socioeconomic impact of the disease.

Key points – allergy: an increasing problem

• Whether a person develops an allergic disease depends on the interaction of risk factors and protective influences.
• Atopic individuals have a genetic predisposition to produce immunoglobulin E (IgE) in response to exposure to small amounts of environmental allergens – this can lead to allergic rhinitis and other atopic disorders.
• Non-atopic individuals can produce IgE, but transiently.
• Increases in the prevalence of allergy have been linked with:
  – decreased rates of infection
  – increased exposure to allergens, pollution and irritants
  – reduced intake of protective nutrients
  – increased stress.

Key references

Bousquet J, Van Cauwenberge P, Khaltaev N. Allergic rhinitis and its impact on asthma. *J Allergy Clin Immunol* 2001;108(5 suppl): S147–334 . www.whiar.org/pocketguide/one.html

Maziak W, Behrens T, Brasky TM et al. Are asthma and allergies in children and adolescents increasing? Results from ISAAC phase I and phase III surveys in Munster, Germany. *Allergy* 2003;58:572–9.

Robinson DS, Larché M, Durham SR. Tregs and allergic disease. *J Clin Invest* 2004;114:1389–97.

Romagnani S. The increased prevalence of allergy and the hygiene hypothesis: missing immune deviation, reduced immune suppression, or both? *Immunology* 2004;112:352–63.

von Hertzen L, Haahtela T. Signs of reversing trends in prevalence of asthma. *Allergy* 2005;60:283–92.

Antigens that elicit an immunoglobulin E (IgE) response are called 'allergens'. Allergenic extracts (e.g. from house dust mites) contain several different molecules. Some of these evoke a response in many people and are termed 'major allergens'. The remainder ('minor allergens') affect only a small proportion of people.

Each allergen molecule comprises a number of antigenic determinants – epitopes. These are small polypeptides recognized by the immune system as being 'non-self'. People vary in their response to different allergen molecules and to different epitopes of the same allergen molecule. As there may be similarities in amino acid sequences between different allergens, cross-reactivity (partial immunologic identity) can occur (e.g. between birch pollen and hazelnut).

Environmental allergens can be quantified: for example, pollens can be sampled in a pollen trap, and mite and animal allergens can be assessed immunochemically from dust collected from a vacuum cleaner. Mold spores can be collected on culture plates and counted. At present, such measures are largely used in epidemiological investigations and research, but they may also be clinically useful, for example in determining exposure at home or work, to be followed by relevant skin-prick tests.

Pollen grains

Pollen grains are the gametes of plants and need to be transferred from one plant to another (Figure 2.1). Insect-pollinated plants usually have bright flowers and produce small numbers of pollens – these rarely cause allergy. Wind-pollinated plants release large quantities of small pollen grains and are the major cause of allergy. As the majority of pollen grains (20–30 µm in size) are trapped in the nose, rhinitis is the usual result. However, pollen allergens released in dew and raindrops have the potential to reach the bronchi as dust, and to cause asthma. This is particularly noticeable during thunderstorms when pollen particles are split into smaller fragments.

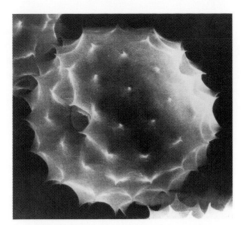

Figure 2.1 Scanning electron micrograph of a grass pollen grain.

Pollen allergy (hay fever or pollinosis) can progress to other forms of sensitization and to more persistent forms of disease. For example, hay-fever sufferers are three times more likely to develop asthma than non-sufferers. There is also a tendency for some to develop persistent rhinitis. This is possibly because, as well as carrying antigens into the respiratory tract, pollen is also a source of bioactive lipids that attract neutrophils and eosinophils, and a source of E phytoprostanes, which inhibit interleukin 12 (IL-12) and modulate dendritic cell function towards T helper 2 (Th$_2$) polarization.

Grass pollen is the most common cause of pollen allergy worldwide – for example, it affects over 95% of people with seasonal allergic rhinitis in the UK. Grasses pollinate in the summer (Figure 2.2). As grass species cross-react extensively, the number of extracts needed for diagnosis and treatment is limited. Bermuda grass (*Cynodon dactylon*), however, is a separate entity.

Pollen is released early in the morning, rises high into the atmosphere and descends in the evening as the air cools. As the pollen season travels northward at about 5° longitude per week, those affected by it may be able to plan a 'pollen avoidance' holiday.

Trees pollinate mainly in the spring; the season is short. In northern Europe, Asia and North America, birch pollen is the main cause of

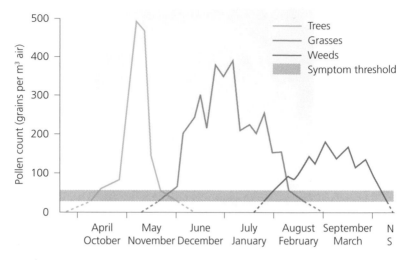

Figure 2.2 The annual calendar of major pollen seasons for trees, grasses and weeds. Most individuals develop symptoms when the pollen count reaches 25–50 grains/m³ air. N, northern hemisphere; S, southern hemisphere.

allergy. It is cross-reactive with hazel pollen and nut, and some people suffer 'birch/apple syndrome', whereby fresh apples and certain vegetables and soft fruit cause oral allergy symptoms (see page 35).

In Mediterranean areas, the olive tree is the major cause of pollen allergy. This is cross-reactive with privet.

Weeds. Ragweed is a major cause of seasonal allergic rhinitis in North America. Its season runs between mid-August and September. Ragweed plants are extensive in grain fields, and ragweed allergy is most prevalent in the midwest region of the USA. The season is later in more southerly areas, in contrast to the grass pollen season.

In Europe, mugwort and *Parietaria* are important weed allergen sources. The latter is a perennial weed found in the Mediterranean basin.

Molds

Molds (microfungi) are microscopic organisms that produce very large numbers of small spores (2–5 µm). These spores can reach the lower airways and thus tend to cause asthma rather than allergic rhinitis.

Molds need conditions of high relative humidity in order to grow: they are prevalent in temperate climates during the late summer, but are present in the tropics in large quantities all year. Molds can be a problem in buildings with damp indoor areas, particularly if disseminated via the air conditioning system. The main pathogens are *Cladosporium*, *Alternaria*, *Aspergillus*, *Penicillium* and *Mucor*.

The extent to which fungal allergy causes rhinitis and rhinosinusitis is a matter of some debate. Fungi are present in nearly all noses, but they are associated with degranulating eosinophils in the nasal mucus in chronic rhinosinusitis, suggesting that fungal hypersensitivity may be an etiologic factor. In fact, this appears unlikely in chronic rhinosinusitis as a whole, since several double-blind placebo-controlled trials have shown no effect of antifungal treatment on symptoms and signs. However, there is undoubtedly one form of rhinosinusitis, allergic fungal sinusitis, in which small quantities of trapped fungi elicit a massive immunologic response (see Antifungal therapy, Chapter 9, page 96).

Animal sources

House dust mites, which are too small to be seen with the naked eye, are the most common indoor source of allergen (Figure 2.3). *Dermatophagoides pteronyssinus* and *Dermatophagoides farinae*, which have strong cross-reactivity, are the most significant species. Other mites such as *Blomia tropicalis*, *Tyrophagus putrescentiae*, *Lepidoglyphus destructor*, *Glycyphagus domesticus*, *Acarus siro* and *Aleuroglyphus ovatus* are more relevant in tropical climates.

The major allergens of the house dust mite are the digestive enzymes Der p1, 2 and 3, and Der f1, which are present in the fecal pellets. These are of similar size to pollen grains and are rendered airborne during dusting and cleaning but settle rapidly (within 30 minutes). Highest exposure to mites occurs during sleep.

Occurrence. Mites require a high relative humidity to survive, as they have no water conservation system. They also breed best at warm temperatures, around 25°C. Ideal conditions exist in mattresses where they have food (human skin scales), warmth and moisture. They also live in carpets, curtains, furniture, pillows, duvets and stuffed toys.

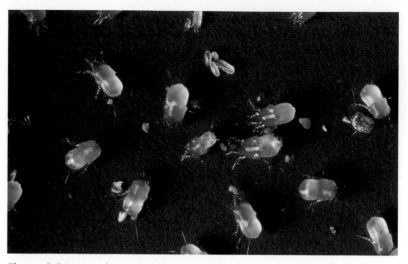

Figure 2.3 House dust mites seen alive with the stereomicroscope. They are the most important cause of perennial allergic rhinitis. Reproduced with the permission of Dr MJ Colloff, Scottish Parasite Diagnostic Laboratory, Stobhill Hospital, Glasgow, UK.

The prevalence of house dust mites in housing has increased over recent decades, reflecting the increasing numbers of energy-efficient, poorly ventilated, centrally heated and carpeted houses.

Mites are a worldwide problem; the only areas relatively spared are deserts with a very dry climate, and high altitudes (above 3000 m).

Storage mites are harbored in stored foods, such as grain in warehouses, granaries and food and farm stores. They are very sensitive to desiccation and are a common cause of allergy in farmers and inhabitants of the tropics, where they are also found in houses. Storage mites do not cross-react with the *Dermatophagoides* species, and extracts of storage mites (*Glycophagus*, *Tyrophagus* and *Acarus*) must be included for adequate allergy investigation in some parts of the world.

Cockroaches. In some inner city areas (e.g. Chicago and New York), a high proportion of people with rhinitis and/or asthma test positive to cockroach extract in skin-prick tests.

Cats and dogs. Over 50% of homes in northern Europe and North America have at least one cat or dog; allergy to these pets is a common cause of symptoms.

In cats, the major allergen (Fel d1) is produced in the salivary glands. Dried saliva in the pelt becomes airborne as small, sticky, allergenic particles. These become attached to carpets, furniture and walls, and remain in the home for about 6 months after the removal of the cat.

In dogs, the major allergens are from the salivary glands, skin scales and urine. Hair itself is not allergenic. The principal canine allergen is Can d1.

Rodents. Hamsters, guinea pigs, mice and rats are popular as pets and are also widely used in medical research. The major allergen occurs in their urine. Atopic subjects commonly become sensitized and react within a year of first exposure.

Horses and cows. Horse allergen is very potent, but most people can easily avoid horses. Cross-reactivity exists between horse dander and the serum used in tetanus vaccine.

Cow allergy is primarily a problem for people who work with cows (e.g. vets, farmers and cowboys). These individuals are, however, still able to eat beef.

Birds. 'Feather allergy' is, in fact, mainly caused by exposure to mites that contaminate feathers. Allergy to bird droppings occurs in people who keep budgerigars or pigeons in poorly ventilated rooms. Bird antigens can cause allergic alveolitis through an IgG mechanism. IgE-mediated allergy, resulting in asthma and rhinitis, is rarely a problem.

Occupational allergens

Rhinitis can be caused by allergens encountered in the workplace and may develop into asthma. Occupational allergens are listed in Table 2.1; they include allergens from small mammals (rats and mice, which can cause rhinitis in laboratory workers), foodstuffs (wheat and pineapple, which can cause problems for bakers and factory workers, respectively),

TABLE 2.1

Major causes of occupational allergic rhinitis

Agent	Allergen	Source
Vegetable proteins	Grains and flour	Food industry, baking
	Latex	Hospital work
Animal proteins	Dander, droppings, fur, urine	Breeding, laboratories
Enzymes (animal and vegetable)	Amylase, cellulase, papain, trypsin	Food industry, detergents, pharmaceuticals, manufacturing
Microbial agents	Antibiotics	Manufacturing, healthcare
Simpler chemicals	Isocyanates, colophony (pine resins)	Plastics, paints, glues, soldering, electrical work
	Acid anhydrides	Epoxy resins

drugs (penicillin can cause responses in healthcare professionals) and latex (healthcare workers). Occupational rhinitis can also be non-allergic (see Chapter 6).

Latex. Small particles of latex attach to the powder in latex gloves and become airborne when gloves are handled, with consequent eye and nose sensitization. Rhinoconjunctivitis is often the first symptom of latex allergy. This can progress to asthma, and latex is a cause of anaphylaxis. The recognition of latex allergy and substitution of non-powdered or non-latex gloves in hospitals has reduced the alarming rise in severe allergy and anaphylaxis caused by latex: an example of allergen avoidance producing significant benefit.

Food allergens

Food allergy is rarely seen in people who have allergic rhinitis but no other symptoms. On the other hand, rhinitis is a common symptom of food allergy in people with multiple organ involvement. Despite the wide variety of foods ingested, only a relatively few foods cause most allergic reactions. In infants under 6 months, the majority of allergic reactions are to egg, milk or soy. In adults, the most common food allergens causing severe reactions are peanuts, tree nuts, fish, crustacea, eggs, milk, soybean, sesame, celery and some fruits, such as apples and peaches.

Key points – allergens

- Pollen allergens cause allergic symptoms when the plants bloom.
- House dust mite allergen is the major indoor allergen in Europe.
- House dust mites prefer warm and humid areas, they feed on human skin scales and prefer to live in beds.
- Cat allergen stays on surfaces and in the air for months after removal of a cat.

Key references

Breiteneder H, Radauer C. A classification of plant food allergens. *J Allergy Clin Immunol* 2004;113: 821–30.

D'Amato G, Spieksma FTM, Bonini S, eds. *Allergenic Pollen and Pollinosis in Europe.* Oxford: Blackwell Scientific Publications, 1991.

Moneret-Vautrin DA, Morisset M. Adult food allergy. *Curr Allergy Asthma Rep* 2005;5:80–5.

The nose acts as an air conditioner that filters, warms and humidifies 10 000 liters of air daily. To accomplish this, it has a specialized structure that incorporates:

- a narrow slit-like orifice
- a large surface area
- mucus and cilia
- a turbulent airflow
- a bend into the nasopharynx (Figures 3.1 and 3.2).

The turbinate bones or conchae, of which there are two or three on each side, cause turbulent airflow so that particles are deposited and can be cleared by the mucociliary system. This moves them to the back of

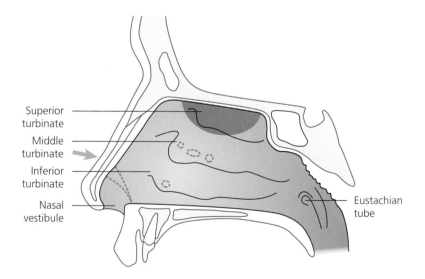

Figure 3.1 Lateral wall of nasal cavity. The arrow points to the internal ostium, and the colored area is the olfactory region. The openings from the naso-lacrimal duct and the paranasal sinuses are under the inferior, middle and superior turbinate.

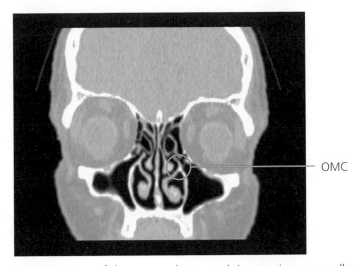

OMC

Figure 3.2 CT imaging of the nose and paranasal sinuses gives an excellent presentation of the anatomy. Note how the mucous membrane in the nose surrounds the bony structures, creating a slit-like air passage. The ostiomeatal complex (OMC) is the site of sinus drainage and ventilation. It is a narrow slit-like orifice easily obstructed by mucosal swelling or thick secretions. Blockage is probably a major factor in the pathophysiology of sinusitis.

the pharynx where they are swallowed. Many particles are deposited on the bend into the nasopharynx. Very few particles larger than 10 µm penetrate further than the nose; particles smaller than 2 µm do not tend to become deposited in the nose. Pollen grains are 20–30 µm in size and tend to cause allergic rhinitis, whereas mold spores, at 2 µm, tend to cause asthma rather than rhinitis. Water-soluble gases, such as sulfur dioxide, formaldehyde and ozone, are retained in the nose and can cause irritation of the nasal mucosa.

The width of the nasal passages is regulated by sympathetic nervous tone that acts on the venous sinusoids. Most individuals have a nasal cycle, with one nostril being more patent than the other for 2–4 hours at a time. This is controlled at brainstem level and is usually inapparent unless a degree of nasal obstruction is present.

Because of its filtration function, the nose is the site of more allergy-related symptoms and illnesses than any other organ.

The paranasal sinuses – which are on each side of the nose, above it and behind it – probably have functions of skull lightening, vocal resonance, shock absorbance and immune defense via production of a microbicidal gas, nitric oxide. Most ventilate and drain into the nose via the ostiomeatal complex – bilateral, slit-like orifices at the level of the nasal bridge (Figure 3.2). Obstruction of the complex by mucosal swelling, polyps or thick secretions is thought to be the initiating factor in rhinosinusitis.

The eustachian tubes enter the posterior part of the nasopharynx and, like the lining of the nose and sinuses, are lined with pseudocolumnar ciliated epithelium. Eustachian tube dysfunction secondary to mucosal edema probably plays a role in the etiopathogenesis of otitis media with effusion.

Olfactory receptors involved in smell perception are situated in the upper part of the nose where minute nerve endings pierce the skull base. Nasal inflammation and obstruction reduces the ability to smell. This is most obviously seen in nasal polyposis, but can occur in other forms of rhinitis.

Allergic inflammation of the nose

This is characterized by the accumulation of T cells, mast cells and eosinophils and occurs in three phases, all of which may occur in the nose at any one time:

- sensitization
- early-phase reaction – mast cell degranulation
- late-phase reaction – inflammation.

Sensitization. Initial contact with allergen at the nasal mucosa, with capture by dendritic cells and presentation to T cells, results in sensitization, with Langerhans' cells acting as antigen-presenting cells. In the atopic individual, the predominant T cell is of the T helper 2 (Th_2) type, producing interleukins IL-3, IL-4, IL-5 and IL-13. In this milieu, the B cells make immunoglobulin (Ig) E rather than IgG. IgE is rapidly and avidly attached to local mast cells (Figure 3.3). This is sensitization. Not all sensitized individuals exhibit clinical symptoms on allergen contact. The reason is unknown, but it

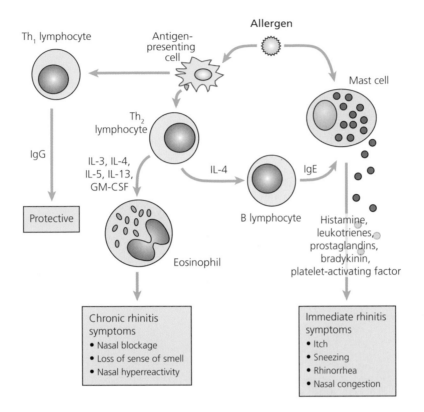

Figure 3.3 Cellular and humoral mechanisms in allergic rhinitis. The recruitment of immune cells from the blood to the nasal mucosa is regulated by adhesion molecules such as intercellular adhesion molecule 1 (ICAM-1). Th$_2$ cells play an important role in orchestrating the inflammatory response by releasing cytokines, including interleukins (ILs) and granulocyte-macrophage colony-stimulating factor (GM-CSF). Mast cells play an important role in immediate symptoms, via the release of histamine and other mediators, while eosinophils contribute substantially to the chronic features of rhinitis.

means testing for IgE, as a sole diagnostic measure can yield false-positive results.

Early-phase reaction. On subsequent exposure, allergen can interact with IgE on the surface of the mast cell causing degranulation and

25

release of mediators, such as histamine. Histamine stimulates sensory nerves and induces reflex sneezing and glandular hypersecretion. It also acts directly on the histamine receptors on blood vessels, causing vasodilatation and edema (Figures 3.4 and 3.5). Antihistamines (H_1 inverse agonists) reduce sneezing and rhinorrhea in people with rhinitis, suggesting that histamine is the major mediator involved in the production of these symptoms. However, antihistamines have relatively little effect on nasal obstruction and hyperresponsiveness where other mediators, such as leukotrienes, bradykinin and eosinophil proteins, are implicated.

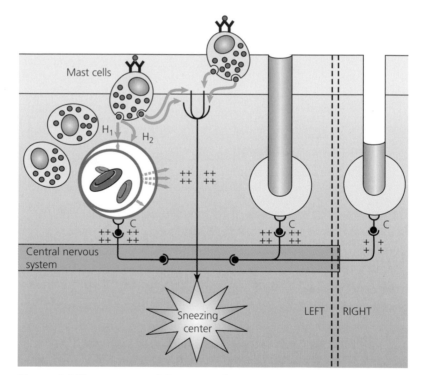

Figure 3.4 The response of the nose to histamine. Histamine acts directly on vascular receptors causing vasodilatation (H_1 and H_2 receptors), plasma exudation and edema formation (H_1 receptors). Histamine stimulates sensory nerves (H_1 receptors) and initiates a parasympathetic reflex via cholinergic receptors (C), which results in hypersecretion in both sides of the nose.

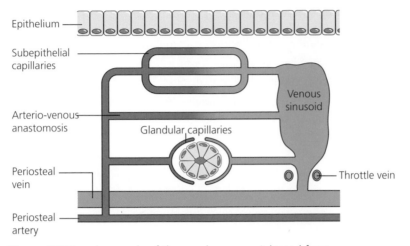

Figure 3.5 Vascular supply of the nasal mucosa. Adapted from Scadding GK. Rhinitis medicamentosa. *Clin Exp Allergy* 1995;25:391–4.

The most recently developed antihistamines (desloratadine and levocetirizine) reduce nasal obstruction demonstrably, possibly via some anti-inflammatory activity related to their ability to inhibit nuclear factor $\kappa\beta$ (a major transcription factor of the inflammatory response).

Late-phase reaction. Some people experience a prolonged or biphasic reaction to allergen contact. This is most commonly seen in people with persistent rhinitis and those exposed to large allergen doses. This phase is associated with an influx of inflammatory cells – mainly eosinophils, but also lymphocytes, mast cells and basophils – under the control of cytokines, such as IL-3, IL-5 and granulocyte-macrophage colony-stimulating factor (GM-CSF), released by Th$_2$ cells, mast cells and local structural cells. The symptoms are nasal obstruction, hyperreactivity to non-specific stimuli and to further allergen contact, and reduced olfaction.

Non-allergic inflammation of the nose

As with intrinsic asthma, there appears to be a form of nasal and sinus inflammation that is similar to that seen in allergy, but which lacks IgE involvement. The major cytokine is IL-5 and eosinophilia is often

27

> ## Key points – pathogenesis
>
> - Allergic rhinitis involves eosinophilic inflammation, which is orchestrated by T cells.
> - The allergic response has an early phase of mast cell degranulation and mediator release with obvious symptoms of sneeze, rhinorrhea and itch.
> - The late phase is less obvious and consists mainly of nasal congestion, which may affect contiguous structures.
> - Non-allergic rhinitis can also involve eosinophilic inflammation without immunoglobulin E.
> - Viral rhinitis often causes sinus inflammation and rarely becomes secondarily bacterial.
> - A certain degree of nasal symptoms is normal.

intense. This is found in NARES (non-allergic rhinitis with eosinophilia), ASA-sensitive respiratory disease (ASA: acetylsalicylic acid, aspirin) and Churg–Strauss syndrome (eosinophilic vasculitis).

Infectious rhinitis. The pathophysiology of rhinoviral infection, the cause of one-third of colds, involves initial attachment of viruses to their receptor, intercellular adhesion molecule (ICAM)-1. This receptor is upregulated in allergy. Attachment begins in the nasopharynx, then the viral infection proceeds to involve the nasal and sinus mucosae. The inflammatory response includes release of bradykinin, which is responsible for some of the swelling, rhinorrhea and discomfort.

Rhinosinusitis can be seen on computed tomography scans for up to 6 weeks after viral infection. Secretions may be discolored, but this does not necessarily imply bacterial infection. The fact that some 0.5–2% of people with viral colds become superinfected with bacteria – usually those same ones that are normally found in the upper respiratory tract (*Staphylococcus* spp., *Streptococcus pneumoniae*, *Haemophilus influenzae*, *Moraxella catarrhalis*) – suggests that the normal immune mechanisms holding these in check have been diminished.

Nervous involvement

Adrenergic fibers in sympathetic nerves cause contraction of blood vessels when stimulated. Consequently, α-receptor agonists (sympathomimetics) are used as nasal decongestants. However, overuse can lead to reduced adrenergic responsiveness and rhinitis medicamentosa (see pages 39 and 75).

Stimulation of the cholinergic fibers involved in parasympathetic nerve transmission causes hypersecretion from submucosal glands that can be inhibited by atropine and ipratropium bromide.

The nasal sensory nerves are constantly being stimulated by pollutants, temperature changes and atmospheric dryness, and there is a constant reflex activity that stimulates mucus production, modulates blood vessel tone and alters nasal patency.

A certain degree of nasal symptoms is normal. It can be difficult to make a clear distinction between a normal physiological phenomenon and rhinitis because individual acceptance of nasal symptoms varies considerably.

Key references

Gelfand EW. Inflammatory mediators in allergic rhinitis. *J Allergy Clin Immunol* 2004;114(5 suppl):S135–8.

Kirtsreesakul V, Naclerio RM. Role of allergy in rhinosinusitis. *Curr Opin Allergy Clin Immunol* 2004;4:17–23.

van Drunen CM, Fokkens WJ. Basophils and mast cells at the centre of the immunological response. *Allergy* 2006;61:273–5.

4   Classification of allergic rhinitis

Allergic rhinitis is clinically defined as a symptomatic disorder of the nose induced by an immunoglobulin E- (IgE)-mediated inflammation after allergen exposure of the membranes lining the nose. Symptoms of rhinitis include rhinorrhea, nasal obstruction, nasal itching and sneezing, which are reversible spontaneously or under treatment.

'Seasonal, perennial and occupational'

Historically, allergic rhinitis has been subdivided, based on the time of exposure, into seasonal, perennial and occupational: perennial allergic rhinitis being most commonly caused by indoor allergens such as dust mites, molds, insects (cockroaches) and animal danders, and seasonal allergic rhinitis being related to a wide variety of outdoor allergens, such as pollens and molds. This classification is not entirely satisfactory for the following reasons.

- Pollens and molds are perennial allergens in some areas (e.g. *Parietaria* pollen allergy in the Mediterranean area).
- Symptoms of perennial allergy may not be present all year round. A large number of individuals allergic to house dust mites only suffer from mild or moderate to severe intermittent rhinitis. This is the case in the Mediterranean area, where levels of house dust mite allergens are low in the summer.
- The majority of individuals are sensitized to many different allergens and are therefore exposed throughout the year: perennial symptoms are often present and individuals present with seasonal exacerbations when exposed to pollens or molds.
- Non-specific irritants, such as air pollution, may aggravate symptoms in symptomatic individuals and induce symptoms in asymptomatic individuals with nasal inflammation.

ARIA classification

In 2001, the World Health Organization (WHO) and other groups put together a working group on rhinitis and its impact on asthma, Allergic

Rhinitis and its Impact on Asthma (ARIA). The document drawn up by the working group proposed a major change in the subdivision of allergic rhinitis, with classification being based on:

- duration, using the terms 'intermittent' and 'persistent'
- severity of symptoms and their impact on social life, school and work, using the terms 'mild' and 'moderate to severe' (Figure 4.1).

Current usage

The terms 'seasonal' and 'perennial' cannot be used interchangeably with 'intermittent' and 'persistent' as they do not represent the same stratum of disease. As most people are polysensitized, it appears that the ARIA classification is closer to the real clinical picture than the previous one.

In western Europe, tree and grass pollens are the most important allergens leading to allergic symptoms in the season. For this reason, 'seasonal allergic rhinitis' is still widely used to describe pollen-allergic rhinitis in spring and summer. Individuals with this are usually more likely to be the 'sneezer' type than the 'blocker' type (see Table 7.4,

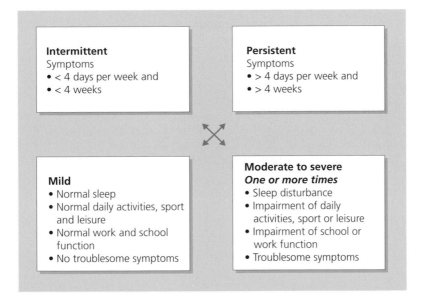

Figure 4.1 Classification of allergic rhinitis according to the Allergic Rhinitis and its Impact on Asthma (ARIA) guidelines. From Bousquet et al. 2001.

31

page 60); there are treatment implications for distinguishing this group, and therefore this term can be retained in addition to the ARIA classification.

Key points – classification of allergic rhinitis

- Allergic rhinitis is a symptomatic disorder of the nose induced by an immunoglobulin E-mediated inflammation after allergen exposure of the membranes lining the nose.
- Allergic rhinitis has historically been subdivided into 'seasonal', 'perennial' and 'occupational', but there are limitations to the usefulness of these terms.
- The Allergic Rhinitis and its Impact on Asthma (ARIA) guidelines use the terms 'intermittent', 'persistent', 'mild' and 'moderate to severe'.
- 'Seasonal' and 'perennial' cannot be used interchangeably with 'intermittent' and 'persistent'.
- 'Seasonal allergic rhinitis' is widely used to describe pollen-allergic rhinitis in spring and summer.

Key references

Bousquet J, Van Cauwenberge P, Khaltaev N. Allergic rhinitis and its impact on asthma. *J Allergy Clin Immunol* 2001;108(5 suppl): S147–334. www.whiar.org/pocketguide/one.html

Johansson SG, Hourihane JO, Bousquet J et al. A revised nomenclature for allergy. An EAACI position statement from the EAACI nomenclature task force. *Allergy* 2001;56:813–24.

Seasonal allergic rhinitis, also known as hay fever, is caused by allergy to pollen grains. In the northern hemisphere, tree pollens cause spring symptoms, grass pollens cause summer symptoms, and in the early fall weed pollens are the causative agent (see Figure 2.2, page 16). Pollen grains are mainly trapped in the nose and also land on the eye, so rhinoconjunctivitis is the major problem. This is sometimes associated with bronchial hyperreactivity or asthma, particularly after thunderstorms.

Seasonal allergic rhinitis has adverse effects on academic performance: in the UK, where 16-year-olds take GCSE mock examinations before the pollen season and take the real examinations in late May or June, hay fever sufferers are 40% more likely than their non-allergic peers to drop a grade from their mock examination mark in English, mathematics or science at GCSE. The 40% figure rises to 70% if sedating antihistamines are used.

Occurrence

About 20% of the population are affected at some time during their lives. The disease usually starts in the childhood or teenage years, with 40% of sufferers noticing symptoms before the age of 6 years. Generally, the earlier the symptoms start the more severe they tend to become. Historically, there was usually a decrease in symptoms by middle age, with very few elderly people being affected. However, a progression from seasonal to perennial rhinitis or rhinosinusitis and to asthma, with the development of further sensitization, is now being observed.

Symptoms

Nasal itch, sneezing and watery rhinorrhea with mild or moderate nasal blockage are the predominant symptoms. Itching of the eyes is also common. Some more severely affected individuals will develop asthma when the pollen count is high. Such people commonly show bronchial hyperreactivity even outside the pollen season.

Symptom severity in the eyes and nose correlates with the pollen count, which is highest in sunny, dry weather. During the hottest part of the day, the pollen rises to 500 m and can travel several miles at that altitude, before descending as the air cools. As a consequence, people in urban areas can be affected.

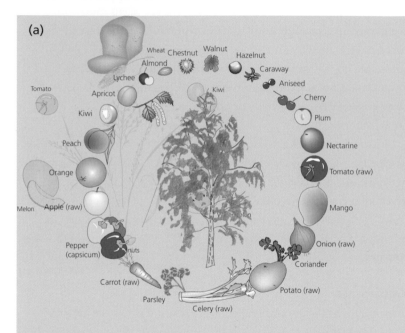

(a)

Figure 5.1 Oral allergy syndrome arises in individuals sensitized to pollens who then cross-react with constituents of the pollen in fresh fruit and vegetables. The reaction usually involves the lips and mouth, with itching and sometimes swelling, but can affect the throat. Usually a person will notice symptoms with one or two foods, rather than all those shown here. The major cross-reacting constituent, profilin, is heat-labile, and therefore cooked fruits are tolerated. (a) Possible cross-reactivity from birch pollen. (b) Possible cross-reactivity from grass pollen. (c) Possible cross-reactivity from latex, derived from the rubber tree.

Oral allergy syndrome. Some pollen-sensitized individuals exhibit cross-reactivity to allergens present in pollen and foods, such as apples, nectarines, cherries, carrots and celery. This is the oral allergy syndrome (Figure 5.1). The symptoms are usually those of itching and swelling of lips and tongue; sometimes the throat is affected, but

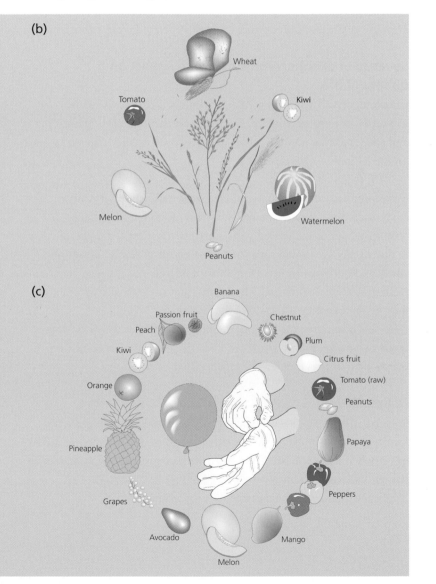

breathing is rarely compromised. Symptoms become more marked during, and for a few months after, the pollen season because of the rise in immunoglobulin E (IgE) that occurs during seasonal exposure. Cooking the food usually destroys allergenicity and prevents symptoms because the relevant proteins are heat-labile. Case study 2 in Appendix III highlights the diagnosis of this syndrome. Similar cross-reactivities are seen in latex-sensitive patients; latex is derived from rubber trees.

Severity of allergic rhinitis based on impact on quality of life

Classic signs and symptoms. Allergic rhinitis is characterized by subjective symptoms (rhinorrhea, nasal obstruction, nasal itching and sneezing) that are difficult to quantify because they depend largely on the individual's perception.

Symptoms associated with social life, work and school. It is now recognized that allergic rhinitis comprises more than the classic symptoms, and is associated with impairments in how people function in day-to-day life. Impairment of quality of life is seen in adults and children. Poorly controlled symptoms of allergic rhinitis may contribute to sleep loss or disturbance. Moreover, sedation with allergic rhinitis may be increased by using sedative treatments.

In several studies, the severity of allergic rhinitis as assessed using quality-of-life measures, work productivity questionnaires and sleep questionnaires was found to be independent of duration.

Diagnosis

Seasonal allergic rhinitis can usually be diagnosed from the person's history, and confirmed by skin-prick or blood testing for specific IgE to grass pollen if needed. See Chapter 7 for more details. The treatment of seasonal allergic rhinitis is covered in Chapter 8. Case study 1 in Appendix III also looks at seasonal allergic rhinitis.

Key points – seasonal allergic rhinitis

- Allergic rhinitis has effects on academic ability.
- Pollen avoidance helps to reduce symptoms.
- Pollen asthma can occur.
- The symptoms can impact on a person's day-to-day life.

Key references

Hellings PW, Fokkens WJ. Allergic rhinitis and its impact on otorhinolaryngology. *Allergy* 2006;61:656–64.

Mari A, Ballmer-Weber BK, Vieths S. The oral allergy syndrome: improved diagnostic and treatment methods. *Curr Opin Allergy Clin Immunol* 2005;5:267–73.

Parikh A, Scadding GK. Seasonal allergic rhinitis. *BMJ* 1997;314: 1392–5.

Chronic rhinitis can roughly be classified into allergic, infectious and non-allergic non-infectious. The exact figures are unknown, but most ear, nose and throat clinics report a 50/50 division between allergic and non-allergic adults with perennial rhinitis.

The disease is non-allergic when allergy has not been proven by proper allergy examination (history, skin-prick testing, measurement of serum-specific immunoglobulin E [IgE] antibodies). Rhinitis is called non-infectious when the nasal discharge is clear and watery and not purulent. Detection of microorganisms (viruses, bacteria, fungi) is generally not used as a diagnostic criterion.

When allergy, mechanical obstruction and infection have been excluded as the cause of rhinitis, a number of poorly defined nasal conditions of partly unknown etiology and pathophysiology remain. The differential diagnosis of non-allergic, non-infectious rhinitis is extensive (Table 6.1). The mechanisms are only partly unravelled. If the pathophysiology is unknown, the term 'idiopathic rhinitis' is used.

Occupation

Occupational non-allergic rhinitis arises in response to an airborne agent present in the workplace. Many occupational agents are irritants and non-allergic hyperresponsiveness may occur. Most agents that cause a reaction are compounds with low molecular weights, such as isocyanates, aldehydes, ninhydrin and pharmaceutical compounds. More than 250 chemical entities have been identified. Although these can act as reactive haptens, non-immunologic mechanisms are common. Some compounds, like chlorine, can induce irritant rhinitis in 30–50% of exposed workers.

Drugs

A range of medications is known to cause nasal symptoms. Reserpine, hydralazine, guanethidine, phentolamine, methyldopa, angiotensin-converting enzyme inhibitors, β-blockers, chlorpromazine, acetylsalicylic

TABLE 6.1

Types of non-allergic, non-infectious rhinitis

- Occupational
- Drug-induced
  - ASA
  - other medications
- Hormonal
- Other causes
  - NARES
  - irritants
  - food
  - emotions
  - atrophy
  - age
- Neurogenic
- Idiopathic

ASA, acetylsalicylic acid; NARES, non-allergic rhinitis with eosinophilia.

acid (ASA) and other non-steroidal anti-inflammatory drugs, oral contraceptives and α-adrenoceptor antagonists such as prazosin have been associated with nasal symptoms, as have intraocular ophthalmic preparations (β-blockers). Psychotropic agents such as thioridazine, chlordiazepoxide, amitriptyline, perphenazine and alprazolam can also have nasal side effects.

Long-term use of topical nasal vasoconstrictors (such as xylometazoline hydrochloride and other α-adrenoceptor agonists) often results in rhinitis medicamentosa with possible histological changes in mucosa, and drug addiction. Rhinitis medicamentosa can be defined as a condition of nasal hyperreactivity, mucosal swelling, rebound nasal congestion and tolerance that is induced, or aggravated, by the overuse of topical vasoconstrictors with or without a preservative. Generally, these individuals can be adequately treated by lucid exposition, vasoconstrictor withdrawal and a topical corticosteroid spray to alleviate the withdrawal process. Occasionally, transient oral corticosteroids may be required. After successful vasoconstrictor withdrawal, any remaining nasal disorder can be treated.

Hormones

Changes in the nose are known to occur during the menstrual cycle, puberty, pregnancy and in specific endocrine disorders such as hypothyroidism and acromegaly. Hormonal imbalance may also be responsible for the atrophic nasal change in postmenopausal women. A persistent hormonal rhinitis or rhinosinusitis may develop during pregnancy in otherwise healthy women. Its severity parallels the blood estrogen level. The symptoms usually disappear quickly after delivery.

Non-allergic rhinitis with eosinophilia syndrome (NARES)

Individuals with NARES complain of sneezing paroxysms, profuse watery rhinorrhea and pruritus of the nasopharyngeal mucosa in an 'on-again-off-again' symptomatic pattern. There is a profound eosinophilia in the nasal smear (more than 25% eosinophils) and no signs of allergy on skin-prick testing and measurement of total and specific IgE in the nasal secretion. It has been suggested that NARES is a precursor of ASA sensitivity. The definition of NARES as a subgroup of non-allergic, non-infectious rhinitis is relevant for therapy because the condition responds well to nasal corticosteroids, in contrast to some other subgroups of non-allergic, non-infectious rhinitis.

Irritants

Smoke, in particular cigarette smoke, is known for its irritative effect on the mucosa of the respiratory tract. A mucosal cellular infiltration is found in non-allergic children exposed passively to smoke and in smoking adults. Because smoking tends to result in many individuals with the same clinical picture of rhinitis with rhinorrhea and nasal obstruction, it has to be viewed as a cause of rhinitis in its own right.

Food

Food allergy rarely causes isolated rhinitis, but in small children egg, milk or other foods can cause a spectrum of symptoms that may include rhinitis as well as gut symptoms, atopic dermatitis, asthma and failure to thrive. Rhinitis also sometimes occurs during anaphylaxis to food.

Gastroesophageal reflux in small children can be associated with cough and nasal discharge.

Food intolerance (in which IgE-mediated mechanisms are not involved) can give rise to nasal symptoms. Histamine-rich foods (cheese, some fish and some wines) may result in flushing, headache and rhinitis, and the same may occur with tyramine-rich foods (bananas). Food additives and coloring agents (e.g. sulfites, benzoates and tartrazine) may also provoke reactions, especially in ASA-sensitive subjects. Finally, alcohol or spicy, hot food containing capsaicin may irritate C fibers and non-specifically provoke rhinitic symptoms.

Occasional patients complain of gustatory rhinitis in which eating any food provokes rhinorrhea. This is probably an autonomic innervation problem and may respond to ipratropium.

Emotions

The nose is extensively innervated and higher centers of the central nervous system input into this network. Honeymoon rhinitis is well described, and stress can cause rhinitis symptoms, or exacerbate other forms of rhinitis.

Atrophic rhinitis

Atrophic rhinitis can occur following radiation exposure or excessive surgery, or in Sjögren's syndrome.

Rhinitis in the elderly

The characteristic clinical picture here is an elderly individual suffering from a persistent clear rhinorrhea without nasal obstruction or other nasal symptoms. Individuals often complain of the classic drop on the tip of the nose.

Autonomic rhinitis

Some patients present with predominant rhinorrhea, especially in the mornings, often associated with nasal hyperreactivity and a tendency to nasal obstruction. An autonomic imbalance with parasympathetic activity overriding the usual sympathetic dominance of the nasal mucosa has been proposed as the cause. Parasympathetic blockade with ipratropium may prove beneficial.

Other neurogenic forms of rhinitis are probable – for example, in association with chronic fatigue syndrome – but elucidation of mechanisms is awaited.

Idiopathic rhinitis

Formerly also called vasomotor rhinitis, idiopathic rhinitis is a diagnosis of exclusion given to individuals suffering from persistent nasal congestion, rhinorrhea and/or sneezing with no identifiable etiology. It is unrelated to allergy, infection, structural lesions, polyposis and other systemic diseases. Histological examination usually shows normal, non-inflamed nasal mucosa. Neurogenic mechanisms have been implicated in some studies; other groups claim that a subset of these individuals has localized allergic disease diagnosable by nasal allergen challenge. The etiology is likely to be mixed.

Key points – non-allergic rhinitis

- Rhinitis is not necessarily an allergic phenomenon.
- Industrial agents and other irritants in drugs, smoke and food can cause rhinitis.
- Hormonal changes and old age are also linked to symptoms.

Key references

van Rijswijk JB, Blom HM, Fokkens WJ. Idiopathic rhinitis, the ongoing quest. *Allergy* 2005;60:1471–81.

Allergy is thought to be the underlying cause of persistent rhinitis in around 80% of children and 30% of adults. Accurate diagnosis is needed for effective treatment.

Taking the history

Assessing the individual's history is the most important part of the rhinitis investigation. The use of a history proforma may be helpful (Table 7.1), not only to save clinic time, but to jog the memories of both individual and investigator so that no relevant fact is omitted. The most important symptom should be noted as this may affect the choice of treatment. The timing of this in relation to the seasons, days, home, pet exposure, work, holidays is noted, together with any relieving factors. Nasal and palatal itching are strongly suggestive of allergy, as is an association with conjunctivitis.

Seasonality. Symptoms occurring exclusively between May and July in the UK are likely to be caused by grass pollen allergy. Individuals often believe that rapeseed (canola) allergy is their problem because the flowers are more obvious and odorous, but rapeseed is rarely the major cause, though the volatile organic compounds it produces may contribute to symptoms. In the southern states of the USA, ragweed pollinates from mid-August to mid-September and is the major cause of seasonal symptoms. However, the continent is so large that climatic variations occur, and tree and grass pollens can also be relevant. Local knowledge is needed for diagnosis.

Duration. The duration of symptoms and their effects on quality of life allows rhinitis to be classified as intermittent or persistent and as mild or moderate to severe according to the ARIA guidelines (see Figure 4.1, page 31; see also Appendix I, page 108). This also has treatment implications.

TABLE 7.1

History for diagnosing rhinitis

Major nasal symptoms (sneezing, itching, rhinorrhea or blockage in order of importance to the individual) and any other associated symptoms affecting ears, sinuses, throat, chest

Timing	• Diurnal variation
	• Effect of holiday
	• Seasonal variation

Provoking and relieving factors

Family history	• Eczema
	• Asthma
	• Rhinitis
	• Urticaria
Past history	• Eczema
	• Asthma
	• Rhinitis
	• Urticaria
Living conditions	• House (age, dampness)
	• Carpets, central heating
	• Bedding
	• Pets
Occupation	• Exposure to allergen and irritants
	• Relation of symptoms to work exposure
Medication	• Present treatment
	• Reactions to medication (e.g. ASA)
	• Use of nasal vasoconstrictors
Diet	• Oral allergy syndrome
	• Other food reactions

ASA, acetylsalicylic acid.

Atopic disease. A past or family history of atopic disease makes an allergic form of rhinitis more likely. Other conditions running in the family (e.g. nasal polyps, infertility, cystic fibrosis, thyroid disease) may also be relevant to the cause of rhinitis.

Environment. A very detailed environmental history – covering feeding, pets, nursery placement, smoking in the home and so forth – may give a clue as to the cause. Many people lead complicated lives and live in at least two places: symptoms occurring at only one can give a clue to causation (e.g. the child whose nose runs at his childminder's house, where there is a dog). Cat dander can be carried to schools and workplaces on the owners' clothes, so sensitive individuals who are not cat owners can still be troubled by cat allergy.

Medication. Any treatments taken for symptoms, including alternative and complementary ones, need to be accurately recorded: how, when and how often they were or are used, together with their effectiveness or otherwise. Other medications, such as antihypertensives and oral contraceptives can cause nasal obstruction, as can overuse of nasal decongestant sprays.

Symptoms at other sites. It is necessary to ask about symptoms at other sites, particularly the lower respiratory tract, ears, skin and gut in small children, and the sinuses and chest in adults.

Emergency signs. The signs of potential complications of infection are shown in Table 7.2. An individual presenting with any of these should be referred immediately.

TABLE 7.2
Emergency signs requiring immediate referral

- Periorbital edema
- Displaced globe
- Double vision
- Ophthalmoplegia
- Reduced visual acuity
- Severe unilateral or bilateral frontal headache
- Frontal swelling
- Signs of meningitis or focal neurological signs

Children. For a child, the history should include details of the pregnancy, birth, postnatal feeding and infections plus development. The child with rhinitis plus atopic eczema and colic may well have food allergies, with milk and egg the most likely causes.

Examination

An individual may show classic allergic features such as a horizontal crease across the nose ('allergic crease'; Figure 7.1a) or give an 'allergic salute', in which the itchy nose is rubbed with the fingers. A double allergic crease (Denny's lines) under the eyes may be noted, and dry, eczematous skin can be apparent (Figure 7.1b). The quiet, withdrawn child may not be able to hear properly.

The skin should be examined for signs of atopic dermatitis, particularly on the face and in the elbow and knee flexures.

Ears, nose and throat. The ears, nose and throat should be examined. An otoscope is useful for all three, but may need to be supplemented by nasal endoscopy (Figure 7.2) if rhinosinusitis is suspected.

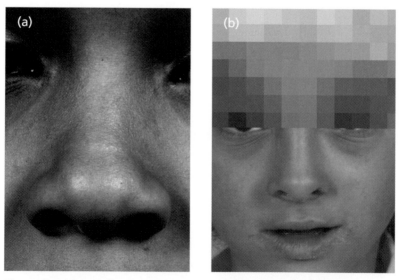

Figure 7.1 (a) An 'allergic crease' visible on a boy's nose. (b) The face of a child shows chronic mouth-breathing, dry eczematous skin and Denny's lines beneath the eyes, all suggesting persistent allergic rhinitis.

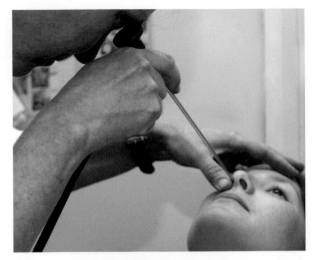

Figure 7.2 Nasendoscopy with a Hopkins rod.

Allergic rhinitis. The classic nasal appearance of allergic rhinitis
involves swollen, pale inferior turbinates and plentiful clear secretions,
but this can also occur in non-allergic rhinitis, and, conversely, the
allergic nose can appear normal or reddened, particularly if topical
corticosteroids have been recently used.

Chronic rhinosinusitis. The mucosa of the nose and sinus are
contiguous and so chronic nasal complaints can also be induced by an
(accompanying) chronic sinusitis (see Chapter 9).

Granulomatous disease. Occasionally other appearances, such as a
septal perforation together with marked crusting and bleeding will
suggest a diagnosis of granulomatous disease, such as Wegener's
granulomatosis or sarcoidosis. Atrophic rhinitis with widely patent,
smelly, crusted nasal mucosa (Figure 7.3) is rarely seen, but can occur
following radiation exposure or excessive surgery or in Sjögren's
syndrome. Polyps may be found. These are distinguishable from
turbinates by their insensitivity, yellow-gray hue and non-attachment to
the lateral nasal wall (see Figure 9.2, page 88).

Chest examination should include observation of chest shape: an
indrawn lower chest suggests an upper airway obstruction. Wheezing
may be audible. The abdomen should be examined if there is any

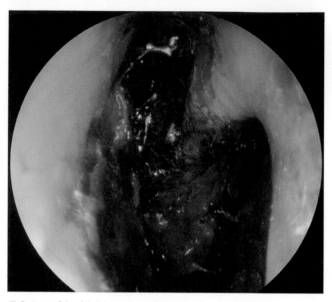

Figure 7.3 Atrophic rhinitis – note the patent, crusted nasal mucosa.

gastrointestinal complaint or if reflux is suspected as a cause of rhinitis symptoms. Clinical signs to look for are shown in Figure 7.4.

Height and weight. The weight and height of children should be recorded. It is sensible to repeat these measurements at each visit, particularly if the child is using topical corticosteroids.

Supplementary tests

A plan for using tests to diagnose rhinitis is given in Figure 7.5. Testing for specific allergies can be undertaken during the clinic visit by skin-prick tests or by taking blood and sending it for laboratory analysis. Allergens should be selected according to the history. Screening for a wide variety of allergens is not recommended as false-positives occur in over 15% of the population, particularly with food allergens.

Skin-prick testing is simple, quick and virtually painless and has a high degree of specificity. A single drop of glycerinated extract is placed on the skin, which is punctured by a 1-mm lancet held at 90° to the skin surface. Precision can be improved if the test is performed in duplicate.

External

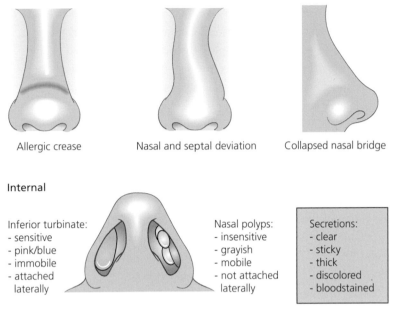

Allergic crease

Nasal and septal deviation

Collapsed nasal bridge

Internal

Inferior turbinate:
- sensitive
- pink/blue
- immobile
- attached laterally

Nasal polyps:
- insensitive
- grayish
- mobile
- not attached laterally

Secretions:
- clear
- sticky
- thick
- discolored
- bloodstained

Check:
ears, throat, chest, neck, skin

Figure 7.4 Clinical signs to look for on examination.

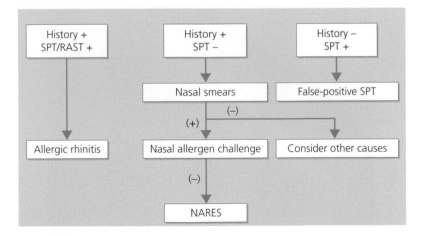

Figure 7.5 Algorithm for testing. NARES, non-allergic rhinitis with eosinophilia; RAST, radioallergosorbent test; SPT, skin-prick test.

49

The test can be undertaken in primary care by a trained operator, provided only inhalant allergens are used. The allergens chosen usually consist of a basic set (house dust mite, grass pollen, cat, dog, plus positive and negative controls) plus any other ones suggested by the history (e.g. other animals, latex, molds). It is advisable to use standardized extracts with consistent potency from a recognized supplier. The strength is usually given in biological units (BU) or in allergy units (AU) per milliliter. When the allergen, introduced into the skin, interacts with immunoglobulin E (IgE) bound to mast cells, it causes histamine release and a consequent 'wheal-and-flare' (edema and erythema) reaction (Figure 7.6).

Controls. A negative control with only the diluent is used to judge the extent of the reaction to the prick procedure itself. This may be large in people with sensitive skin (dermographism). A positive control with histamine is used to judge skin reactivity and to discover whether there is any interfering antihistamine medication.

Safety. Although skin-prick testing practically never causes problems, it is sensible to have epinephrine available.

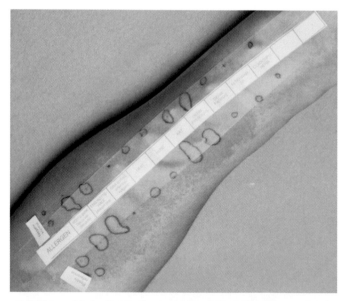

Figure 7.6 Skin-prick testing is the most important allergy examination. A positive test gives a 'wheal-and-flare' reaction.

Influencing factors. Antihistamines and some antidepressants depress skin reactivity, so treatment must be stopped 4 days before testing. Dermal corticosteroids also reduce reactivity, though systemic corticosteroids do so only in high doses (about 30 mg per day). Individuals with widespread eczema or dermographism and those with previous anaphylaxis should have blood rather than skin-prick tests.

Reading the reaction. The maximum histamine reaction occurs at 10 minutes, and the allergen reaction occurs at 15 minutes. A reaction site with diameter 3 mm bigger than the negative control is usually taken to be positive (Figure 7.7). If a permanent record is required, the wheal can be outlined by felt-tip pen and the markings transferred to squared paper by means of tape.

Skin-prick testing must be interpreted in light of the individual's history. A positive skin-prick test can occur in a symptom-free person (latent allergy), but this indicates an increased risk of later symptom development (tenfold in the case of grass pollen). For a symptomatic individual, exposure to allergen causing a positive skin-prick test will usually be of clinical significance. However, the test will remain positive years after symptoms have disappeared and after immunotherapy.

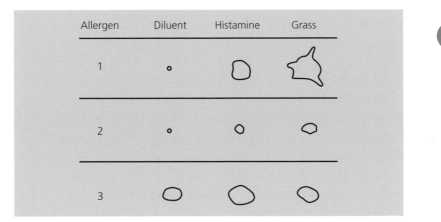

Figure 7.7 Reading a skin-prick test for allergy to grass pollen. 1 = A clear positive test with the pollen reaction larger than the positive control with histamine; 2 = a false-negative test with a very small reaction to histamine caused by use of an oral antihistamine before testing; 3 = a false-positive test in an individual reacting to the diluent (dermographism).

Aero-allergen skin-prick test reactivity correlates well with symptoms. This is not the case for food allergens, where false-positive skin-prick test reactions often occur. The best way to diagnose food allergy is by dietary exclusion and re-introduction. Attempts to diagnose food allergy in a person with isolated symptoms of rhinitis will very rarely lead to clinical benefit.

Measurement of specific IgE. The RAST (radioallergosorbent test) was the first laboratory test for allergen-specific IgE in serum (Figure 7.8). The more recent version (CAP System, Phadia AB, Uppsala, Sweden) has increased sensitivity.

The advantages of blood testing include absolute safety, standardization, a high degree of precision, independence from medication and lack of side effects (such as causing increased itching in people with eczema). The disadvantages include high cost and lack of immediately available results.

The measurement of specific IgE is no more sensitive than skin-prick testing. It can be used when skin-prick testing is unavailable or inadvisable, such as in people taking antihistamines or those with severe atopic dermatitis. It can also be used as a supplement to skin testing where there is doubt regarding the clinical significance of the result and when a confirmatory test is needed (e.g. before immunotherapy).

Total serum IgE. Normal values of IgE vary widely with age, and there is a considerable overlap between atopic and non-atopic individuals. Most people with isolated rhinitis have a normal IgE level. However, total serum IgE is a valuable test when used thoughtfully in selected people with rhinitis plus asthma.

Elevated levels of IgE also occur in atopic dermatitis, allergic bronchopulmonary aspergillosis and worm infestations.

Blood eosinophil count. The degree of blood eosinophilia depends on the size of organ affected by allergy. Consequently, blood eosinophils are raised in atopic dermatitis and asthma, but are rarely elevated in isolated rhinitis. The eosinophil count is generally higher in perennial non-allergic rhinitis than in allergic rhinitis.

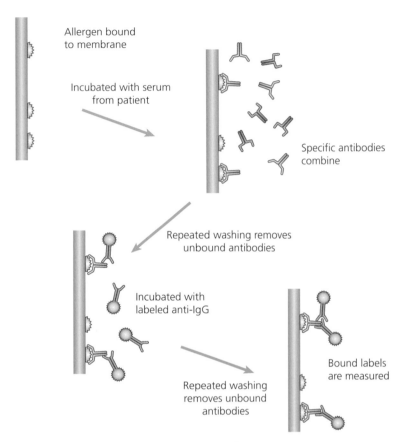

Allergen bound
to membrane

Incubated with serum
from patient

Specific antibodies
combine

Repeated washing removes
unbound antibodies

Incubated with
labeled anti-IgG

Repeated washing
removes unbound
antibodies

Bound labels
are measured

Figure 7.8 Measurement of allergen-specific immunoglobulin E with the radioallergosorbent test.

Blood eosinophils are also elevated in:
- infestation with parasitic worms
- polyarteritis nodosa
- Hodgkin's disease
- Loeffler's syndrome
- Churg–Strauss syndrome
- hypereosinophilic syndrome
- many skin disorders
- drug allergy
- bronchopulmonary aspergillosis.

Nasal smears are most reliably taken using a Rhinoprobe (Arlington Scientific, Arlington, TX, USA) or a similar device. Smears should be taken from both sides of the nose by running the probe along the inferior turbinates two or three times and then smearing the results onto a clear glass slide and fixing them. Slides can be stained with Giemsa to show eosinophils. Other cells, such as neutrophils and squamous cells, and the presence of bacteria can be readily identified (Figure 7.9). There is no consensus as to the definition of nasal eosinophilia, with authorities quoting from 5% to 25% eosinophils being necessary for the diagnosis.

This time-consuming test is infrequently used, but can help to differentiate between allergic rhinitis and repeated common colds in children and in people with negative skin-prick tests in whom non-allergic rhinitis with eosinophilia (NARES) is a possibility. Like blood eosinophilia, nasal eosinophilia, though seen in allergic rhinitis, is usually more marked in people with nasal polyposis in whom skin-prick testing is usually negative. In rhinitis the presence of eosinophils in a nasal smear suggests an inflammatory form of rhinitis. Nasal eosinophilia also predicts a good response to topical corticosteroids. In asthma, the sputum eosinophil count, which varies with disease severity, is a useful guideline for treatment, particularly for corticosteroid requirement. Corticosteroids reduce eosinophilia.

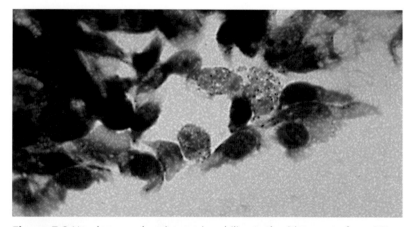

Figure 7.9 Nasal smear showing eosinophilia. Authorities quote from 5% to 25% eosinophils for a diagnosis of nasal eosinophilia.

Allergen nasal challenge. Recent work has suggested that in some people with negative skin-prick tests, IgE may be localized to the nasal mucosa. The diagnosis of allergic rhinitis can be made by nasal provocation with the likely allergen, with some objective measures of nasal response such as rhinomanometry, acoustic rhinometry or nasal inspiratory peak flow, together with symptom scores. This is a procedure for the specialist rhinology clinic, as occasionally subjects develop severe symptoms such as asthma.

ASA nasal challenge. Individuals with rhinitis and/or nasal polyps who are negative to skin-prick tests should be asked about adverse reactions to acetylsalicylic acid (ASA) and non-steroidal anti-inflammatory drugs (NSAIDs). Two well-characterized reactions involving rhinoconjunctivitis, asthma, urticaria or angioedema are diagnostic. Many people, however, will not have taken any recent ASA or NSAIDs but could still be reacting to similar substances in foods and food additives. The diagnosis is then made in a specialized center by ASA challenge.

Lysine ASA is the only truly soluble form of ASA. It is useful for establishing the diagnosis of ASA-sensitive nasal polyposis or rhinitis. Nasal challenge has a high specificity and sensitivity (Table 7.3) and, provided a small dose – for example 8 mg – is used, it very rarely causes lower respiratory tract problems. The time course of the response is delayed, with symptoms starting at around 45 minutes to 1 hour. This

TABLE 7.3

Sensitivity and specificity of ASA challenge according to route

	Challenge sensitivity (%)	Challenge specificity (%)
Oral	77	93
Bronchial	77	93
Nasal	73	94

ASA, acetylsalicylic acid.
Lysine ASA, the only completely soluble form, must be used for nasal or bronchial challenges; in the UK it is not easily available and has to be imported.

contrasts with allergen challenge, in which sneezing is almost immediate and nasal obstruction is established within 15–20 minutes.

Nasal airway tests may be needed to establish that objective nasal obstruction exists (as the dry, widely patent nose also feels blocked). They can also be useful for establishing the response to nasal challenges as described above. If used before and after nasal decongestant, the degree to which mucosal swelling compromises the airway can be established, together with the need for any structural alteration to the nose such as turbinate reduction or septal surgery.

Different methods exist:
- nasal inspiratory peak flow
- nasal expiratory peak flow
- anterior rhinomanometry
- posterior rhinomanometry
- acoustic rhinometry
- lower airway tests
- nitric oxide levels.

Nasal inspiratory peak flow measurement uses a peak-flow meter with an anesthetic mask attached. The individual is asked to exhale completely, then to close their mouth. The mask is fitted tightly over the nose and mouth; care must be taken not to deform the nose and to establish a tight seal. The person then inhales deeply and suddenly as hard as possible. Three readings are usually taken and accepted if the variation is less than 10%. A few people are unable to perform this successfully; others find it distinctly uncomfortable. However, if able, the person can take the machine home to carry out serial recordings and test the effect of environmental exposure or response to medication.

Nasal inspiratory peak-flow measurements have been shown to correlate with those obtained by rhinomanometry.

Nasal expiratory peak flow measurement is difficult and messy and is rarely used.

Anterior rhinomanometry uses a flow monitor in one nostril while resistance is simultaneously measured. It is technically demanding, and it can be difficult to obtain consistent results in many people, particularly those with marked nasal blockage or neurogenic rhinitis.

Posterior rhinomanometry. Here, the monitor is placed in the posterior nasopharynx. The results are more accurate and reproducible than those achieved with anterior rhinomanometry, but some 20% of people are unable to tolerate the procedure.

Standardized conditions for rhinomanometry have been described.

Acoustic rhinometry sends a train of five acoustic clicks into the nose and records the echoes with a microphone. The information is Fourier-transformed by a computer and expressed as a graph of the nasal area versus distance into the nose. This method is quick, results are obtainable in most noses and reproducibility is good in the anterior part of the nose. Consensus guidelines for performance of acoustic rhinometry exist.

Lower airway tests. In view of the frequent concurrence of asthma with rhinitis it has been recommended that all people with persistent rhinitis should undergo lower airway testing for possible asthma.

Peak flow is the simplest test. A peak-flow meter is used to record three forced expirations and the best result is noted. A nomogram can be used to decide if this is within normal limits for the individual's age, sex and height. The test can be repeated following administration of a bronchodilator or following exercise. The person can also be asked to undertake recordings at home and return with a peak-flow chart. A diurnal variation of more than 20% suggests asthma.

Spirometry is similar, but involves a forced expiration, which is continued until the person cannot exhale any further (Figure 7.10). Again, three values are recorded and the forced expiratory volume in 1 minute (FEV_1) is noted, together with the forced vital capacity. The ratio between the two gives a measure of lower airway patency, with most people achieving over 80%. Lower values suggest obstruction.

This test can be performed before and after bronchodilator administration to assess the degree of reversibility of lower airway obstruction.

Nitric oxide levels. The measurement of nitric oxide (NO) in the airways has been largely restricted to the laboratory (Figure 7.11).

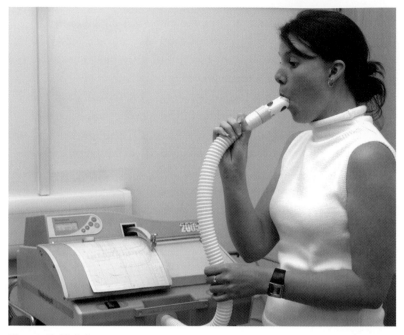

Figure 7.10 Spirometry.

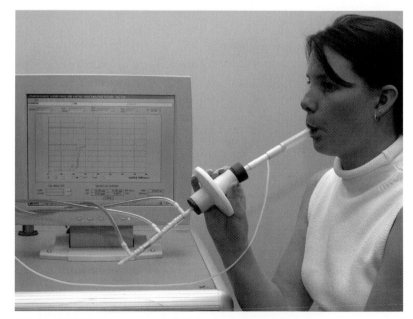

Figure 7.11 Measurement of nitric oxide in the airways.

However, the fact that air exhaled from the lungs usually contains less than 20 ppb NO unless inflammation is present gives a means of identifying lower airway inflammation. The cause of an elevated exhaled NO (eNO) is not identified and it can be infection-related or inflammatory. In asthma, eNO levels correspond to sputum eosinophilia, and rises in eNO usually precede asthma exacerbations, so such levels are under investigation as a means of directing asthma therapy.

In the nose, the situation is more complex because the sinuses continuously produce high levels of NO (around 20–25 ppm), probably as a defense against bacteria, fungi and tumors. NO from the sinuses normally passes into the nose via the ostiomeatal complexes. In addition, nasal mucosal NO production can be induced in response to infection or inflammation. Thus, nasal NO (nNO) levels are a composite of nasal mucosal production and sinus production. High levels of nNO suggest an inflammatory rhinitis. Very low levels can occur either in response to sinus obstruction (chronic rhinosinusitis, nasal polyposis) or to failure of production (primary ciliary dyskinesia). In the latter, extremely low levels (< 100 ppb) are often found in the nose. These do not rise in response to decongestants or to a course of oral steroids. In this instance, subsequent investigations of cilia by ciliary beat frequency assessment and electron microscopy should be undertaken.

Children with cystic fibrosis tend to have low nNO levels. They also can have nasal polyps, which should prompt sweat tests and genetic tests for cystic fibrosis.

Making the diagnosis

Allergic rhinitis can usually be diagnosed from the person's history, confirmed by skin-prick or blood testing for specific IgE to the allergen if necessary.

Allergic rhinitis is classified as either intermittent or persistent, and mild or moderate to severe according to the ARIA guidelines (see Figure 4.1, page 31). In addition, those with allergic rhinitis broadly fall into two groups: 'sneezers and runners' and 'blockers' (Table 7.4). Identifying the group into which an individual falls can help guide therapy.

TABLE 7.4

Distinguishing 'sneezers' from 'blockers' with allergic rhinitis

Symptom	Sneezers and runners	Blockers
Sneezing	• Especially paroxysmal in bouts	• Little or none
Rhinorrhea	• Always present: watery, anterior and sometimes posterior	• Variable, can be thick mucus, and generally more posterior
Nasal itching	• Yes, often	• No
Nasal blockage	• Variable	• Often severe
Diurnal rhythm	• Worse on awakening, improves during the day and usually worsens again in the evening	• Constant day and night, may be worse at night and is often severe
Conjunctivitis	• Often present	• None

All those with persistent rhinitis should be examined and tested for asthma and other lower respiratory tract problems.

Non-allergic rhinitis. To exclude all known prevailing causes of chronic rhinitis, a full history should be taken (medication, smoking in previous 6 months, occupation, etc.), commonly occurring inhalation allergies should be excluded (by skin-prick testing and/or specific serum IgE measurement) and anterior rhinoscopy and nasendoscopy should be used to exclude gross anatomic aberrations and nasal polyps.

If chronic rhinosinusitis is obvious on examination (polyps, mucosal edema or discharge at the middle meatus), computed tomography (CT) is unnecessary. This is also the case where the history and nasendoscopy do not suggest possible sinus problems (see Chapter 9 for more information on the diagnosis of rhinosinusitis). CT scans should only be used where there is diagnostic doubt, particularly if sinister signs, such as unilateral symptoms or blood-stained discharge, are present.

Case studies

Four case studies are included in Appendix III. They look at the diagnosis and/or treatment of:

- seasonal allergic rhinitis
- oral allergy syndrome
- recurrent otitis media with effusion
- a child with a runny nose.

Key points – diagnosing rhinitis

- The history is most important – a proforma may be helpful.
- External examination of the nose may reveal an allergic crease or salute.
- Internal nasal examination can be achieved using an otoscope.
- Typically, someone with allergic rhinitis has swollen, pale inferior turbinates and plentiful clear secretions.
- The nose may appear normal in allergic rhinitis.
- All persistent rhinitis sufferers should be examined and tested for asthma or other lower respiratory tract problems.
- Skin-prick or blood tests for allergy can substantiate the history.
- If negative, other causes of rhinitis should be considered.

Key references

Board of Directors. American Academy of Allergy and Clinical Immunology. Allergen skin testing. *J Allergy Clin Immunol* 1993;92: 636–7.

Clement PA. Committee report on standardization of rhinomanometry. *Rhinology* 1984;22:151–5.

Dreborg S, Frew A. Position paper: allergen standardization and skin tests. *Allergy* 1993;48(suppl 14): 48–82.

Hilberg O, Pedersen OF. Acoustic rhinometry: recommendations for technical specifications and standard operating procedures. *Rhinol Suppl* 2000;16:3–17; *Rhinol* 2001;39:119.

Reid MJ, Lockey RF, Turkeltaub PC, Platts-Mills TA. Survey of fatalities from skin testing and immunotherapy 1985–1989. *J Allergy Clin Immunol* 1993;92:6–15.

Scadding G. Nitric oxide in the airways. *Curr Opin Otolaryngol Head Neck Surg* 2007;15:258–63.

Scadding GK et al. BSACI Rhinitis management guidelines 2007. *Clin Exp Allergy* 2007;in press.

Treatment of rhinitis depends on the diagnosis; it broadly falls into:

- allergen avoidance
- pharmacotherapy
- immunotherapy
- surgery
- patient education.

Allergen avoidance

Although it is not practicable to avoid allergen exposure completely (Figure 8.1), the allergen load can usually be reduced. In principle, this is the first measure for a person with allergic rhinitis to take, particularly when the individual is a child. Allergen avoidance is thought to reduce the need for drug therapy and may reduce the risk of progression to asthma, though this has not been proved.

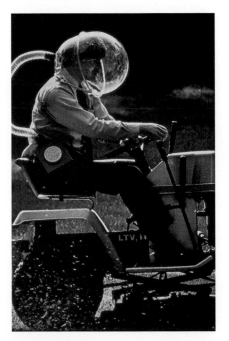

Figure 8.1 Although allergen avoidance is, in principle, the first step in allergic rhinitis therapy, it is not always feasible.

House dust mite. Avoidance measures are advised, particularly in
the bedroom (Table 8.1). Reducing a high indoor humidity, though
difficult, can help to decrease the number of mites, but double-blind
trials have failed to show major clinical efficacy. No trial has yet looked
at multiple methods of allergen avoidance.

Pets. Avoiding pets is easy, in principle at least. However, people do
not always follow the advice. Family pets should be kept out of
bedrooms at all times, but this measure alone is not sufficient as most
pets, particularly cats, are a source of potent allergens that are light and
become distributed throughout the home. It may take months after the
animal has been removed for the full benefit to be felt.

TABLE 8.1

**Evidence for the effectiveness of house dust mite avoidance
measures in the bedroom**

Measure	Evidence in favor	Evidence against
Cover mattresses and pillows with plastic or allergen-impermeable covers	–	A
Wash bed linen at > 55°C and damp-wipe mite-proof covers every 1–2 weeks	D	–
Have linoleum or wooden flooring instead of carpet	D	–
Use acaricides on carpets and soft furnishings	–	–
Remove all unnecessary dust-collecting items	D	–
Remove soft toys	D	–
Use leather, plastic or vinyl furniture rather than upholstered furniture	D	–
Do not dry clothes on radiators or store unused clothing in the bedroom	D	–

A = evidence from meta-analysis or more than one double-blind placebo-
controlled trial; D = expert opinion

Superheated steam cleaning can denature all protein allergens and may be beneficial.

Indirect exposure from animal protein on other people's clothes – for example, in schools – cannot be avoided. This can cause problems in highly sensitive individuals.

Pollen exposure leads to more inflammation in the nose, which leads to more symptoms on further exposure. Many people do not understand this and a simple explanation is often helpful.

Allergen exposure can be reduced by avoiding areas where there is likely to be a lot of pollen, such as grassland, and by going out in the middle of the day when pollen is high in the air, rather than early morning or evening when it is rising and descending, respectively. Car windows should be kept closed and a filter installed on the air intake. Showering and washing hair after pollen exposure may help to prevent further symptoms.

Bedroom windows should be closed in the early evening – some firms provide fitted screens that allow air through but exclude pollen. Washed bed linen hung out to dry should be brought in before it becomes coated with pollen in the evening.

Planning of holiday timetables so that the sufferer is by the sea or abroad at the height of the pollen season can reduce symptoms.

Nasal air filters are now available over the counter – these are inserted into the nostrils at the start of the day and are worn continuously all day (Figure 8.2). They significantly reduce nasal symptoms, but not everyone can tolerate them.

Mold avoidance is difficult, but improving ventilation and reducing humidity may help, as may applying bleach to the affected areas of the home.

Nasal washing

Normally the nose cleans itself adequately using the mucociliary apparatus. However, mucociliary function is impaired during infection and in chronic rhinitis. Nasal douching using an isotonic solution (one teaspoon – 5 mL – of salt in 500 mL of water), is particularly

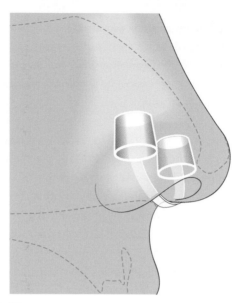

Figure 8.2 Nasal air filters.

beneficial in chronic infectious rhinosinusitis and seasonal allergic rhinitis in young children. It can also alleviate nasal dryness. The simplest method is to pour some into the palm of the hand and sniff it up the nose. Alternatively, squeezable nasal douching bottles, syringes or a saline spray can be employed.

Pharmacotherapy

The drugs available for use in rhinitis are:
- corticosteroids (topical, oral)
- antihistamines (topical, oral)
- cromoglicate
- vasoconstrictors
- cholinoceptor antagonists
- antileukotrienes.

Evidence in favor of their use for allergic rhinitis is excellent (Table 8.2). A recent analysis of the risks and benefits of these drugs is summarized in Table 8.3.

Figure 8.3 summarizes the Allergic Rhinitis and its Impact on Asthma (ARIA) guidelines for treating allergic rhinitis.

TABLE 8.2

Evidence levels supporting pharmacotherapeutic agents and allergen avoidance for allergic rhinitis

Intervention	Seasonal allergic rhinitis		Perennial allergic rhinitis	
	Adult	Child	Adult	Child
Oral antihistamines	A	A	A	A
Intranasal antihistamines	A	A	A	A
Intranasal corticosteroids	A	A	A	A
Intranasal cromoglicate/nedocromil sodium	A	A	A	A
Subcutaneous immunotherapy	A	A	A	A
Sublingual/nasal immunotherapy	A	A	A	A
Allergen avoidance	A	D	D	D

A = evidence from meta-analysis or more than one double-blind placebo-controlled trial; D = expert opinion. Note: Level A evidence exists against the use of allergen-proof bed covers in isolation.
Adapted from Bousquet et al. 2001. www.whiar.org/pocketguide/one.html

Topical corticosteroids can be first-line therapy in moderate to severe hay fever, adult perennial allergic rhinitis, idiopathic (non-allergic) rhinitis and nasal polyposis. These agents reduce inflammation by reducing inflammatory cell infiltration and the production of pro-inflammatory cytokines. The anti-inflammatory action improves nasal airflow, particularly in the case of allergy. The new generation of nasal corticosteroid preparations has strong local anti-inflammatory effects and very low or negligible systemic side effects. They come as sprays, powders and/or drops. Regular use results in improved nasal airflow and olfactory function, and reduced rhinorrhea. Meta-analysis has shown that intranasal corticosteroids are the most effective medication presently available for the treatment of allergic rhinitis and some types of idiopathic

TABLE 8.3

Benefits and risks of various treatments for allergic rhinitis

Treatment	Benefit	NNT	Harm	NNH	TT
Antihistamine (class mean)	0.066	15.2	0.02	51	23
Nasal steroids (class mean)	0.229	4.4	0.021	48	0.08
Nasal antihistamines					
• azelastine (daily)	0.16	6.3	0.031	32	0.16
• azelastine (twice daily)	0.2	5	0.046	22	0.19
Montelukast	0.07	14.3	0.006	167	0.08
Omalizumab	0.081	12.3	0.08	13	0.50
Immunotherapy	0.218	4.6	0.072	14	0.25

NNH, number needed to harm (the number of patients who must be treated to cause one case of harm); NNT, number needed to treat (the number who must be treated to prevent one adverse outcome); TT, treatment threshold (the probability of disease above which the patient should be treated, 1/[benefit/risk + 1]).
Adapted from Portnoy JM, Van Osdol T, Williams PB. Evidence-based strategies for treatment of allergic rhinitis. *Curr Allergy Asthma Rep* 2004;4:439–46.

rhinitis (Figure 8.4). Their major limitations are a relatively slow onset of action and the lack of effect on eye symptoms.

This treatment can be used once daily, which helps with concordance. For idiopathic rhinitis, topical spray once or twice daily, preferably combined with nasal saline lavage, 0.9%, should be tried for a minimum of 6 weeks before evaluation, as it can take a few weeks to reach the maximum treatment effect (often symptoms can respond after longer-term use when short-term treatment has apparently failed).

There do not seem to be any major differences between the modern corticosteroid molecules (e.g. beclometasone dipropionate, flunisolide, budesonide, fluticasone propionate, triamcinolone acetonide, mometasone furoate) in terms of efficacy.

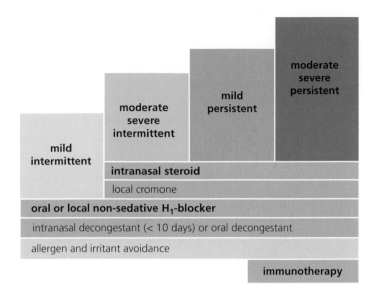

Figure 8.3 Allergic Rhinitis and its Impact on Asthma (ARIA) guidelines for the treatment of allergic rhinitis. Adapted from Bousquet et al. 2001.

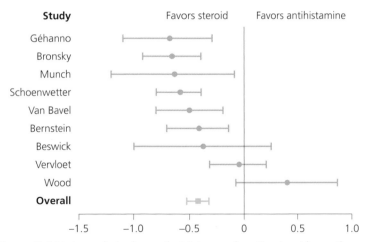

Figure 8.4 Meta-analysis shows that intranasal corticosteroids are the most effective medication presently available for the treatment of allergic rhinitis and some kinds of idiopathic rhinitis. Reproduced with permission from Weiner JM, Abramson MJ, Puy RM. Intranasal corticosteroids versus oral H_1 receptor antagonists in allergic rhinitis: systematic review of randomised controlled trials. *BMJ* 1998;317:1624–9.

Bronchial hyperreactivity, which occurs with seasonal allergic rhinitis in some individuals, can be reduced by nasal treatment with corticosteroids.

Side effects. There is a degree of systemic absorption from the nose, but systemic side effects are not a problem at routine doses in adults. Initial sneezing and irritation may occur, largely owing to nasal hyperreactivity, but these effects should decrease with time. Dryness and bloodstained crusting in the anterior part of the nose occur in around 10% of individuals, but these effects can be reduced by proper use of the spray so that it does not impinge on the same point of the septum every time (Figure 8.5). If epistaxis occurs and is severe, stopping the

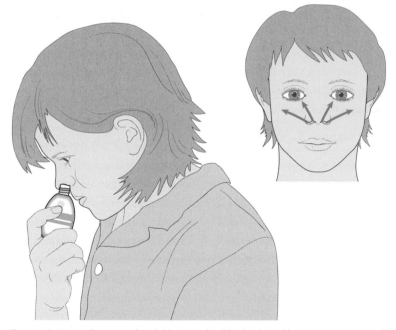

Figure 8.5 Nasal sprays should be used with the head leaning downwards. Using the hand opposite the nostril to be sprayed, two applications are made in different directions towards the outer wall of the nose, thus avoiding septal deposition and epistaxis. This is then repeated on the opposite side of the nose. The individual should be encouraged not to sniff the spray hard into the nose, but to allow it to remain in situ, as it will then be propelled by nasal mucociliary clearance from the front to the back of the nose over 10–20 minutes, during which time it exerts its effect.

spray for a few days, using ointment in the nose and changing the formulation may help.

Corticosteroid sprays have been around for 25 years, and there is no risk of atrophic rhinitis with long-term use. Rarely, a septal perforation can develop.

Children. Intranasal glucocorticosteroids are the most effective treatment of allergic rhinoconjunctivitis, but the fear of systemic side effects, albeit extremely rare, should always be considered in children. The modern intranasal glucocorticosteroids are much less absorbed by the body than the older formulations. The minimal dose needed to control symptoms should be used. Intranasal glucocorticosteroids with high bioavailability, such as betamethasone, should not be used in children. Recent studies have shown that modern corticosteroids such as fluticasone and mometasone have no effect on growth or growth velocity in contrast to oral and depot corticosteroid preparations, which have clear effects.

Pregnancy. No medication, including intranasal steroids, is considered 100% safe during pregnancy, particularly during the first trimester. Obviously the risk–benefit ratio for any prescription must be assessed but, in general, topical agents are preferable to systemic ones, and an established treatment is preferable to a new one.

Oral antihistamines. First-generation H_1-receptor antagonists were developed from tranquilizers and all caused some degree of sedation or psychomotor impairment. The sedating antihistamines, such as chlorphenamine and diphenhydramine, reduce academic performance in children and should therefore no longer be used to treat rhinitis (Figure 8.6). These drugs have now been replaced by second-generation H_1 blockers, which are non-sedating or marginally sedating. These include loratadine, cetirizine, acrivastine, ebastine, fexofenadine, mizolastine, desloratadine and levocetirizine.

Pharmacology. These drugs are rapidly absorbed from the gastrointestinal tract, and onset of effect occurs within 1 hour. They are almost all metabolized by the hepatic cytochrome P450 system. Cetirizine and levocetirizine are exceptions, being excreted unchanged in the urine; fexofenadine is metabolized to a small extent. Most drugs

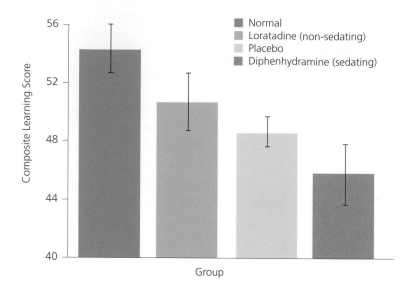

Figure 8.6 Children with seasonal allergic rhinitis learn less well than those without. Their performance is improved by a non-sedating antihistamine, but worsened by a sedating antihistamine. The composite learning score was obtained by a computer program about farming in the desert; children scored higher the longer they maintained their farm by providing water and food. Reproduced with permission from Vuurman EF, van Veggel LM, Uiterwijk MM. Seasonal allergic rhinitis and antihistamine effects on children's learning. *Ann Allergy* 1993;71:121–6.

are effective in a single daily dose, giving good concordance; acrivastine needs to be taken three times daily.

Clinical effects. Although effective against eye and nasal itching, sneezing and nasal running, these agents have only a little effect on nasal blockage. They are more effective in seasonal allergic rhinitis than in perennial disease, where blockage is a greater problem. Regular use has been shown to be more effective than use 'as needed'. This is probably because the histamine receptors exist in equilibrium between two forms: activated and inactive. Antihistamines stabilize the inactive form (i.e. they are inverse agonists). Once treatment is stopped there is a switch back to the active form, with consequent exacerbation of symptoms.

Side effects. Diphenhydramine, terfenadine and astemizole can all block potassium channels and, if blood levels are raised, cause prolongation of the cardiac QT interval, leading to serious ventricular tachycardia. This can occur after overdoses, where liver disease impairs drug metabolism or when drugs such as ketoconazole or erythromycin, or grapefruit juice, are competing for hepatic metabolism. It is also more likely if there are pre-existing cardiac problems or low potassium levels. The potential for an antihistamine to have this side effect is shown in Table 8.4.

Sedation depends on the ability of an antihistamine to cross the blood/brain barrier and react with central or cerebral histamine H_1 receptors. There is still a degree of sedation in some individuals with second-generation antihistamines; this is probably lowest with fexofenadine.

Topical antihistamines. The recent development of topical antihistamines for use in the eyes and nose has meant that itching and sneezing can be quickly relieved without risk of systemic side effects. The major preparations currently available are levocabastine and azelastine, which can be given twice daily or on an 'as-needed' basis. The major side effect with azelastine is taste disturbance.

Two double-blind placebo-controlled trials have shown a therapeutic effect for azelastine nasal spray in people with idiopathic rhinitis with nasal obstruction and/or rhinorrhea. The precise mode of action (antihistaminic, anti-inflammatory or otherwise) remains to be elucidated.

Systemic corticosteroids. In severe cases, a short course of systemic corticosteroids can quickly reduce intranasal inflammation and lead to symptom relief, which can then be maintained with topical corticosteroids. Treatment is short-term (1 week or less), and courses should not be taken more frequently than every 3–6 months. In principle, systemic corticosteroids are not used instead of other treatments, but in addition to a basic medication.

Prednisolone or prednisone, 0.5 mg/kg/day, can be taken orally. Depot injections can cause tissue atrophy at the injection site, cannot be

73

TABLE 8.4

Cardiac effects of antihistamines*

Not seen	Only at very high concentrations	At moderately high concentrations
Cetirizine	Loratadine	Diphenhydramine
Fexofenadine		Hydroxyzine
Desloratadine		Terfenadine
		Astemizole
		Desmethylastemizole
		Norastemizole
		Mizolastine
		Ebastine
		Azelastine

*Antihistamine blockade of the K^+ channels encoded by *HERG1* can, rarely, result in life-threatening ventricular arrhythmias.

removed if side effects occur and are not temporally suited to seasonal disease, as they are most effective when first given, whereas hay fever tends to worsen with duration. Depot injections of steroid into swollen nasal turbinates or polyps have been reported to cause blindness in a few individuals and must, therefore, be avoided.

The major areas of systemic corticosteroid use are:
- at the start of treatment if nasal obstruction is severe
- in the pollen season when counts are very high.

Contraindications include glaucoma, herpetic keratitis, diabetes mellitus, severe hypertension, advanced osteoporosis, peptic ulcer, psychic instability and active tuberculosis. Systemic steroids should not be used for rhinitis in children, or during pregnancy.

Cromoglicate and nedocromil sodium have weak activity in terms of symptom relief and must be administered twice to four times daily. They are both poorly absorbed and virtually free from side effects. Cromoglicate is available as a nasal spray and as eye drops, nedocromil as eye drops. The major area of use is for perennial allergic rhinitis in young children.

Topical vasoconstrictors/decongestants. α-adrenoceptor agonists cause blood-vessel constriction and therefore decongest the nose. They are best given intranasally.

Onset of action is quick and, in the cases of xylometazoline and oxymetazoline, prolonged (6–8 hours). However, people like these sprays and tend to overuse them. These agents do have a place in treatment:

- at the start if the nose is very congested
- during the obstructive phase of colds and sinusitis
- in acute otitis media to relieve ear pain
- when flying if eustachian tube dysfunction is a problem.

They have a very limited role in the therapeutic arsenal of chronic idiopathic rhinitis. Regular, long-term use can result in rhinitis medicamentosa, in which there is rebound nasal congestion and hyperreactivity. Use must, therefore, be restricted to 1 week.

Oral vasoconstrictors/decongestants. Although less effective than topical agents, the oral formulations are not associated with rhinitis medicamentosa.

Unfortunately, the dose needed to treat a stuffy nose is at the borderline with that causing systemic side effects, such as restlessness, difficulty in sleeping, tachycardia, palpitations, tremor and hyperactivity (children). Oral vasoconstrictors are not suitable for people with hypertension, coronary disease, prostatism, thyrotoxicosis, glaucoma or diabetes mellitus. They must not be used at the same time as monoamine oxidase inhibitors. Combined preparations of α-agonists (which can relieve nasal blockage) and antihistamines (which can relieve itching, sneezing and rhinorrhea) are available, but are no more effective than antihistamine alone after the first few days.

Cholinoceptor antagonists. Isolated watery rhinorrhea that is not associated with itch or sneezing rarely responds to the approaches outlined previously. However, as watery discharge is mediated via cholinergic receptors in the nasal glands, antagonists of these receptors are effective. Ipratropium bromide is available as a nasal spray. It is useful for watery rhinorrhea in isolation and rhinorrhea induced by hot, spicy food or exposure to cold air, and it can be helpful in the common cold. It is also the first option for rhinitis of the elderly.

The nasal spray can be used four to six times a day initially. The dose needs to be adjusted for symptom severity and timing (most people experience rhinorrhea in the mornings). The number of doses per day can usually be decreased once control is established. The major side effect is nasal dryness, which can be alleviated by a saline spray. Dry mouth, urinary retention and glaucoma are occasional side effects.

Antileukotrienes. To date, montelukast and zafirlukast are available in the UK, and zileuton, montelukast and pranlukast are available in the USA. These relatively new drugs are effective when taken orally for both asthma and rhinitis. They have efficacy similar to that of antihistamines in the treatment of rhinitis.

Use of combined antileukotriene and antihistamine showed a statistical improvement compared with either one as monotherapy in large trials, but the differences were small and the benefit is unlikely to be clinically relevant in many individuals.

There appears to be a spectrum of responsiveness to antileukotrienes, with around 50–60% of people experiencing some benefit and 10% experiencing marked benefit. Antileukotrienes can be particularly helpful for relieving nasal blockage and restoring the sense of smell. At present, antileukotrienes have a role in treating seasonal rhinitis in people with asthma.

Capsaicin. Repeated administration of capsaicin (five treatments of intranasal capsaicin on a single day at 1-hour intervals, after local anesthesia) leads to a significant and long-term reduction of symptoms in people with idiopathic rhinitis. However, capsaicin is not readily available and its use is restricted to selected centers.

Immunotherapy

Allergen-specific immunotherapy (allergen vaccination) comprises regular subcutaneous injections of allergen in a formulation designed to reduce allergic sensitization and consequently reduce symptoms in the nose, eyes and chest. It is most effective where there is a single, well-defined allergen such as in hay fever.

Indications. Immunotherapy is effective in people suffering from pollen, animal and, to a lesser extent, mite allergy (Figure 8.7). There is some evidence that immunotherapy alters the natural history of allergic diseases, with reduction of progression to asthma in children, together with a reduction in further sensitization.

Before immunotherapy can be considered, the individual must:
• be diagnosed with a skin-prick test or radioallergosorbent test
• have a history of symptom exacerbation on exposure to the particular allergen.

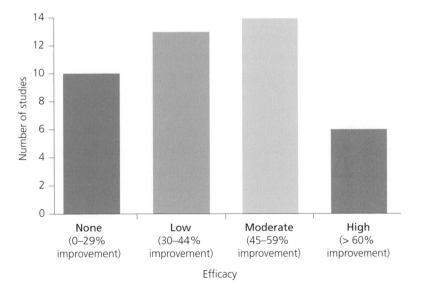

Figure 8.7 Studies showing the efficacy of immunotherapy in patients suffering allergy (all types). Reproduced with permission from Malling HJ. Immunotherapy as an effective tool in allergy treatment. *Allergy* 1998;53:461–72.

Young adults and children over 5 years of age are probably the best candidates for such treatment; in the elderly, the results are less impressive and side effects more common.

Chronic asthma is a contraindication to immunotherapy in the UK.

Pollens. Controlled studies have shown efficacy with grass, birch, ragweed, mugwort, *Parietaria* and cedar in the treatment of rhinoconjunctivitis and asthma. People with severe rhinitic symptoms not controlled by pharmacotherapy should be considered for immunotherapy, particularly if the allergen season is long.

Animal proteins. Avoidance is the major mode of treatment for these individuals, but occasionally this is impossible (e.g. farmers, vets, laboratory workers or school children exposed to pet dander on the clothing of their classmates). Immunotherapy may be useful for these individuals, but it should not be a substitute for allergen avoidance.

House dust mite. Controlled trials in adults have not shown definite efficacy with house dust extracts, though studies in children have. Immunotherapy may be tried in young people who still have severe rhinitis symptoms despite mite avoidance measures and symptomatic therapy.

Contraindications. People with severe asthma or with a significant irreversible airway disease (forced expiratory volume in 1 minute [FEV_1] < 70%) should not be given immunotherapy because of the risk of serious allergen-induced bronchoconstriction. The ideal candidate is a young person with severe rhinitis and either no or mild asthma.

Good compliance is vital and those individuals who cannot attend regularly or who are alcohol or drug abusers should not be included on an immunotherapy program. Other serious risk factors are the presence of cardiovascular disease and the use of β-blockers.

Mechanism of action. The efficacy of immunotherapy is thought to relate to downregulation of T helper 2 (Th_2) responses, with a switch to either Th_1 or Th_0 responsiveness (Th_0 cells produce cytokines that are characteristic of both the Th_1 and Th_2 responses). There is evidence that T cell suppression and cytokines such as interleukin 10 (IL-10) may be involved in this (Figure 8.8).

Extracts. Only one or, at most, two allergens should be used, based on the results of allergy testing, knowledge of allergens in the person's local environment and the potential for avoidance.

High-quality, standardized allergen extracts with little batch-to-batch variation should be used. Aqueous extracts require many injections and cause frequent systemic reactions. Depot extracts, in which aluminum hydroxide or tyrosine has been used to alter the nature of allergen, cause delayed absorption; fewer injections are required and the risk of systemic reaction is reduced.

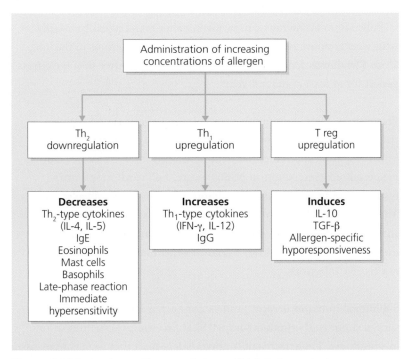

Figure 8.8 Mechanisms of immunotherapy. IFN, interferon; Ig, immuno-globulin; IL, interleukin; TGF, transforming growth factor; Treg, regulatory T cell (or suppressor T cell).

Technique. Immunotherapy has two phases:
- increasing dose
- maintenance.

With depot preparations, the first phase comprises weekly injections, while maintenance injections are 6–8 weeks apart. During the increasing-dose phase, the dose is doubled with each injection if the preceding injection has caused little reaction. If there is a large local reaction or a systemic reaction, either the same dose is given again or a lower dose is given and the doses are increased more slowly. The optimal dose for maintenance injections is the highest dose tolerated without serious side effects. This must be given at regular intervals, and a strict safety regimen must be followed (see below).

With an aqueous extract, rush desensitization can be undertaken with the individual hospitalized to receive 2–6 injections daily over 1 week.

Pollen immunotherapy can be given either pre-seasonally, usually with weekly doses, or perennially, requiring few injections in the long term. The duration of treatment is usually 3 years. After this, the effects persist for at least another 4 years.

Precautions. Every immunotherapy injection is associated with a risk of systemic allergic reaction, such as anaphylaxis or severe bronchospasm. Therefore, the treatment is given by trained operators in specialized centers, not in primary care. Full cardiorespiratory resuscitation facilities must be to hand, together with epinephrine. The individual must be observed for at least 30 minutes following each injection (1 hour in the UK). Those with an asthma episode or those who are suffering from a cold or other systemic illness should not receive injections.

Sublingual immunotherapy. Studies conducted in Europe have shown sublingual immunotherapy (SLIT) to confer some reduction in symptoms. The effectiveness appears less than that of subcutaneous immunotherapy, but the treatment is much safer, with no severe side effects being reported. It is also possible for the treatment to

> **Key points – therapeutic principles**
>
> - The principles of allergen avoidance should be explained to a person with allergic rhinitis.
> - Intranasal corticosteroids are the most effective pharmacotherapy for allergic rhinitis and some types of idiopathic rhinitis.
> - Sedating antihistamines and injected depot corticosteroids are not recommended.
> - Treatment should be started early and continued regularly in moderate to severe intermittent allergic rhinitis.
> - Immunotherapy is effective for very severely affected individuals whose allergic rhinitis is not controlled by pharmacotherapy.
> - Surgery should be considered only for those people who do not get symptomatic relief with medical therapy.
> - Good-quality patient education is helpful.

be taken at home after medical supervision of the first dose. Large double-blind placebo-controlled trials have recently reported results: treatment with grass pollen tablets showed a mean reduction in symptoms of 30% and a 38% mean reduction in the need for medication during the first year of treatment. The long-term effects of 3 years' continuous treatment are under investigation.

Surgery

Surgery should be considered only for those people who do not get symptomatic relief with medical therapy. Surgery in allergic rhinitis patients is usually performed in order to establish a nasal airway into which local treatment can be delivered. Surgical procedures for non-allergic, non-infectious rhinitis aim mainly to modify the size of the inferior turbinate or to reduce septal deviation if obstruction is a problem (Figure 8.9). The reported duration of effectiveness varies from 6 months to several years.

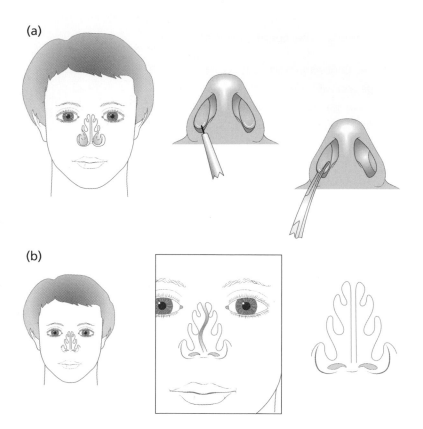

Figure 8.9 Nasal surgery. (a) Turbinate reduction: part of the inferior turbinate is removed to increase patency. However, if too much is removed the patient can develop symptoms of atrophic rhinorrhea. (b) Septoplasty: if the nasal septum is deviated, nasal patency can be reduced. The septum can be straightened surgically.

Patient education

In any chronic disease where the individual needs to take long-term therapy it is vital to explain:

- the nature of the disorder and its possible complications
- why medication is needed
- how medication works
- how and when to use medication
- the likely side effects.

Providing a contact point (telephone or internet) is sensible so that further questions can be asked if the person finds this necessary. Explanatory videos and leaflets in the clinic are helpful and people should be provided with details of useful websites and organizations. All these measures are likely to improve concordance.

Case studies

Four case studies are included in Appendix III.

Key references

Bousquet J, Lund VJ, van Cauwenberge P et al. Implementation of guidelines for seasonal allergic rhinitis: a randomized controlled trial. *Allergy* 2003;58:733–41.

Bousquet J, van Cauwenberge P, Aït Khaled N et al. Pharmacologic and anti-IgE treatment of allergic rhinitis: ARIA update (in collaboration with GA2LEN). *Allergy* 2006;61:1086–96.

Bousquet J, Van Cauwenberge P, Khaltaev N. Allergic rhinitis and its impact on asthma. *J Allergy Clin Immunol* 2001;108(5 suppl): S147–334.
www.whiar.org/pocketguide/one.html

Durham SR. Treatment of seasonal allergic rhinitis: desensitisation for hay fever works. *BMJ* 2003;327: 1229.

Durham SR, Walker SM, Varga EM et al. Long-term clinical efficacy of grass-pollen immunotherapy. *N Engl J Med* 1999;341:468–75.

Fokkens W. Outpatient therapy for nonallergic rhinitis. *Clin Allergy Immunol* 2007;19:363–73.

Nelson HS. Advances in upper airway diseases and allergen immunotherapy. *J Allergy Clin Immunol* 2004;113:635–42.

Schenkel EJ, Skoner DP, Bronsky EA et al. Absence of growth retardation in children with perennial allergic rhinitis after one year of treatment with mometasone furoate aqueous nasal spray. *Pediatrics* 2000;105:E22.

Terreehorst I, Hak E, Oosting AJ et al. Evaluation of impermeable covers for bedding in patients with allergic rhinitis. *N Engl J Med* 2003;349:237–46.

Till SJ, Francis JN, Nouri-Aria K, Durham SR. Mechanisms of immunotherapy. *J Allergy Clin Immunol* 2004;113:1025–34.

Van Rijswijk JB, Boeke EL, Keizer JM et al. Intranasal capsaicin reduces nasal hyperreactivity in idiopathic rhinitis: a double-blind randomized application regimen study. *Allergy* 2003;58:754–61.

Wilson DR, Lima MT, Durham SR. Sublingual immunotherapy for allergic rhinitis: systematic review and meta-analysis. *Allergy* 2005; 60:4–12.

Yáñez A, Rodrigo GJ. Intranasal corticosteroids versus topical H_1 receptor antagonists for the treatment of allergic rhinitis: a systematic review with meta-analysis. *Ann Allergy Asthma Immunol* 2002;89:479–84.

Definitions

Acute rhinosinusitis is defined as sudden onset of two or more symptoms, one of which should be either nasal blockage/congestion or nasal discharge, plus:

- facial pain/pressure and/or
- reduction/loss of smell.

Symptoms last for less than 12 weeks.

Common cold/acute viral rhinosinusitis is defined as acute symptoms of rhinosinusitis for less than 10 days. Children have six to ten common colds per year, adults usually two or three. The most usual causative agents are rhinovirus (> 50%), coronavirus (15–20%), respiratory syncytial virus (RSV) and parainfluenza virus. Infection with the influenza virus (flu) usually causes a more severe acute rhinosinusitis, which is also characterized by high fever and malaise. This is more likely than other infections to result in complications and high-risk groups need pre-seasonal flu vaccination according to national guidelines.

Hand washing can reduce transmission of the relevant viruses.

Acute non-viral (bacterial) rhinosinusitis is defined as acute symptoms of rhinosinusitis for less than 12 weeks, with symptoms increasing after 5 days or symptoms persisting for more than 10 days. The most common cause is bacterial infection, of which *Streptococcus pneumoniae* (20–35%) and *Haemophilus influenzae* (5–25%) are the most common infecting organisms. However, a range of others, including *Moraxella catarrhalis*, *Staphylococcus aureus* and anaerobic bacteria, can also cause symptoms.

Chronic rhinosinusitis with or without nasal polyps is defined as inflammation of the nose and the paranasal sinuses characterized by two or more symptoms, one of which should be either nasal blockage/congestion or nasal discharge, plus:

- facial pain/pressure and/or
- reduction/loss of smell.

Symptoms last for more than 12 weeks.

Nasal polyps and chronic rhinosinusitis are often treated as one disease entity because it seems impossible to differentiate them clearly. Nasal polyposis is considered a subgroup of chronic rhinosinusitis.

Pathophysiology and etiology

Acute rhinosinusitis. The pathophysiology of rhinoviral infection is addressed on page 28.

Chronic rhinosinusitis without polyps. The predisposing factors here include innate and acquired immune deficiency. Often, however, no underlying predisposition can be identified. Biofilm infection may feature in the pathogenesis; this is currently under investigation. In a biofilm, bacteria exist in colonies protected by alginate – this renders the immune system and antibiotics ineffective.

The role of allergy in sinus disease is still unclear. It has been speculated that nasal inflammation induced by immunoglobulin E (IgE)-mediated mechanisms favors the development of acute and/or chronic sinus disease. A similar inflammation is observed in the nose and sinuses of people with allergic rhinitis. Moreover, computed tomography (CT) has revealed sinus involvement in allergic individuals during the ragweed pollen season, and a sinus reaction following nasal challenge with allergen. However, at present it remains incompletely understood whether and via which mechanisms the presence of allergic inflammation in the nose predisposes the individual to the development of sinus disease.

Epidemiological studies are inconclusive and, so far, there are no published prospective reports on the incidence of infectious rhinosinusitis in populations with and without clearly defined allergy. Several epidemiological studies report a high prevalence of sensitization to inhalant allergens in individuals with acute and chronic rhinosinusitis. The prevalence ranges up to 84% of those undergoing revision sinus surgery. One may not, however, conclude that allergic rhinitis predisposes to the development of chronic rhinosinusitis on the basis of epidemiological studies, as these studies have a large referral bias. A predominance of allergy to persistent versus intermittent allergens was found in individuals with chronic sinusitis at the time of indication for surgery. Moreover, epidemiological studies failed to demonstrate a higher incidence of sinus disease during the pollen season in pollen-sensitized individuals.

Nasal polyps. The question remains as to why 'ballooning' of mucosa develops in some but not all people with rhinosinusitis. Nasal polyps have a strong tendency to recur after surgery, even when aeration is improved. This may reflect a distinct property of the mucosa of certain individuals which has yet to be identified. Nasal polyps appear as grape-like structures in the upper nasal cavity, originating from within the ostiomeatal complex (Figures 9.1 and 9.2). They consist of loose connective tissue, edema, inflammatory cells and some glands and capillaries, and are covered with varying types of epithelium, mostly respiratory pseudostratified epithelium with ciliated cells and goblet

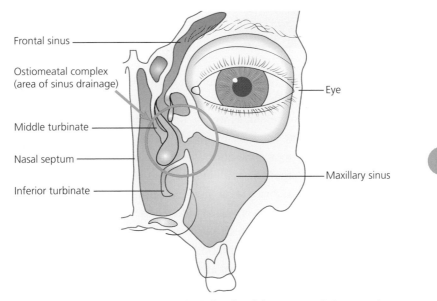

Figure 9.1 Cross-section through the left side of the nose and sinuses. The ostiomeatal complex is highlighted. This area is of the utmost importance for sinus pathology as it contains the openings to the paranasal sinuses. Its function is compromised by nasal polyps, which form in the middle meatus.

87

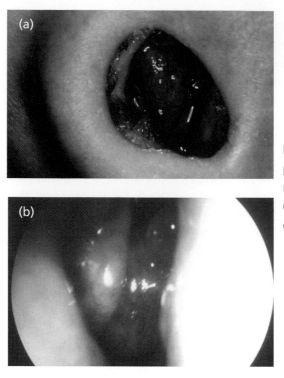

Figure 9.2 Nasal polyps: (a) visible at nasal entrance; (b) visible only on endoscopy.

cells. Eosinophils are the most common inflammatory cells in nasal polyps, but neutrophils, mast cells, plasma cells, lymphocytes and monocytes are also present, as well as fibroblasts.

There is a definite relationship in people with 'Samter's triad' – asthma, sensitivity to non-steroidal anti-inflammatory drugs (NSAIDs) and nasal polyps – though not all individuals with NSAID sensitivity have nasal polyps, and vice versa. In the general population, the prevalence of nasal polyps is 4%. In individuals with asthma, a prevalence of 7 to 15% has been noted whereas nasal polyps are found in 36–60% of people with NSAID sensitivity.

It had long been assumed that allergy predisposed to nasal polyps because the symptoms of watery rhinorrhea and mucosal swelling are present in both diseases, and eosinophils are abundant. However, epidemiological data provide no evidence for this relationship: polyps are found in 0.5–1.5% of people with positive skin-prick tests for common allergens.

Diagnosis

When diagnosing rhinosinusitis, exclude possible allergic causes by asking about allergic symptoms (i.e. sneezing, watery rhinorrhea, nasal itching and itchy, watery eyes). Skin-prick tests or specific IgE measurement should be performed if there is doubt.

Individuals with nasal polyps who are skin-prick test negative should be asked about adverse reactions to acetylsalicylic acid (ASA) and NSAIDs as ASA/NSAID hypersensitivity may be present but undiagnosed, particularly in those with late-onset asthma. This hypersensitivity cannot be diagnosed by skin-prick testing as it is not IgE-mediated, but nasal challenge with lysine ASA, followed by oral challenge if negative, can be used (see page 55).

Emergency signs of potential complications of infection are shown in Table 7.2, page 45.

Chronic rhinosinusitis. If a child has chronic symptoms of rhino-sinusitis, consider primary ciliary dyskinesia and cystic fibrosis. In the case of an adult with chronic symptoms, consider acquired immune deficiencies such as common variable, infective (HIV) and iatrogenic (steroids, immunosuppressants) immune deficiencies and chronic organ failure (e.g. kidneys, liver).

When diagnosis is based on symptoms only, the disease is likely to be overestimated. Nasal endoscopy is preferable and CT imaging is warranted for those with serious or refractory symptoms.

Endoscopic signs include:
- polyps and/or
- mucopurulent discharge from the middle meatus and/or
- edema/mucosal obstruction primarily in the middle meatus.

CT scans may be necessary for an accurate diagnosis. However, the correlation between a CT scan and the severity of rhinosinusitis symptoms is low to non-existent. Roughly one-third of unselected adults and 45% of unselected children have abnormal CT scans, probably because changes persist for 6 weeks following a common cold. Therefore, CT scans of sinuses should be ordered only in secondary care and only then for individuals with sinister symptoms or signs, or those with endoscopically diagnosed chronic rhinosinusitis that is not responding after at least 6 weeks of medical treatment. CT scans of individuals with chronic rhinosinusitis show mucosal changes within the ostiomeatal complex and/or sinuses.

Allergic fungal rhinosinusitis is diagnosed according to strict criteria (Table 9.1). Diagnosis of fungal hypersensitivity is difficult for the following reasons. Molds are often ubiquitous and spore intermittently when atmospheric conditions are correct. Thus, symptoms may be intermittent and difficult to ascribe to any particular cause. Mold extracts for allergy testing are poorly characterized and tend to be derived from the parent plant rather than the spores, which contain the allergens likely to cause symptoms. Extracts may contain mitogens which non-specifically stimulate T cells.

Treating acute rhinosinusitis

Acute rhinosinusitis is usually a self-limiting (viral) infection, though bacterial superinfection can arise. Symptoms due to inflammation of the contiguous nasal and sinus mucosal membrane can last from several days to as long as a few weeks. Even bacterial rhinosinusitis is often a self-limiting disease and more than 70% of people spontaneously recover within 14 days. Treatment can, in most cases, be symptomatic, using nasal saline lavages, decongestants and pain relievers.

Reviewers from a Cochrane group concluded that for acute maxillary sinusitis confirmed radiographically or by aspiration, current evidence is

TABLE 9.1

Criteria for the diagnosis of allergic fungal rhinosinusitis

- Polypoid chronic rhinosinusitis
- IgE-mediated hypersensitivity to fungi
- Heterogeneity, expansion or erosion seen on CT scan
- Eosinophilic mucin, but no fungal invasion into soft sinus tissue
- Fungi in sinus contents on smear

CT, computed tomography; IgE, immunoglobulin E.
Adapted from Bent JP III, Kuhn FA. Diagnosis of allergic fungal sinusitis. *Otolaryngol Head Neck Surg* 1994;111:580–8.

limited but supports the use of penicillin or amoxicillin for 7 to 14 days. Clinicians should weigh the moderate benefits of antibiotic treatment against the potential for adverse effects. There are no indications that antibiotics with a broader spectrum have a more beneficial effect. Given the increasing prevalence of antibacterial-resistant respiratory pathogens, concern is growing about the overuse of antibiotics.

Recently, nasal corticosteroids as monotherapy or in addition to antibiotics have been shown to be effective. In the monotherapy study, nasal corticosteroid was more effective than amoxicillin.

Applying local zinc gel at the start of a cold may reduce its severity and duration, as may altering nasal pH.

A treatment scheme for acute rhinosinusitis is shown in Figure 9.3.

Treating chronic rhinosinusitis with or without nasal polyps

Pharmacological treatment is the cornerstone of treatment for chronic rhinosinusitis with or without nasal polyps. Treatment is aimed at reducing inflammation and infection and restoring ciliary function and mucosa aeration. The choice of treatment is influenced by many factors: past medication, symptom duration, allergy, the presence of polyps and an increased prominence of purulent rhinorrhea on nasal endoscopy. A management scheme for chronic rhinosinusitis is shown in Figure 9.4.

Nasal washing. Conservative treatment should start with simple measures. Nasal secretions present on the nasal mucosa are harmful for several reasons: they impair nasal ciliary function and mucosal aeration and they contain bacteria and cytotoxic cell debris that can cause even more inflammation. Moreover, symptoms of postnasal drip, rhinorrhea and decreased nasal airflow result from the accumulation of nasal secretions in the nasal cavity. Nasal washings are recommended – nasal lavage with isotonic (NaCl 0.9%) or hypertonic saline solutions (NaCl 3.5% or 5%) has been shown to improve quality of life and endoscopic manifestations in a Cochrane meta-analysis.

Corticosteroids. Local corticosteroids are the first choice of medication. They reduce inflammation by reducing inflammatory cell infiltration and the production of pro-inflammatory cytokines. Corticosteroids

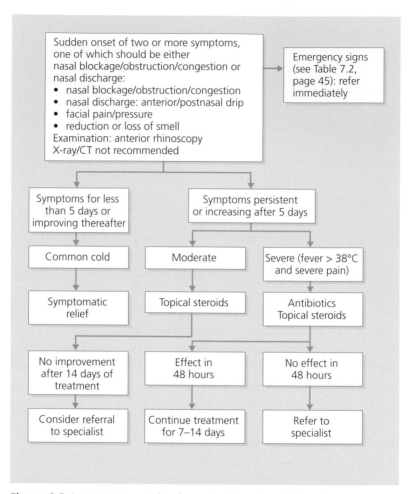

Figure 9.3 A management plan for acute rhinosinusitis in primary care. Adapted from European Position Paper on Rhinosinusitis and Nasal Polyps (EP3OS). *Rhinol Suppl* 2007;20:1–139, with permission (www.rhinologyjournal.com/EPOS2007.pdf).

have strong anti-inflammatory effects and improve nasal airflow, particularly in the case of allergy. The new generation of nasal corticosteroid preparations have strong local anti-inflammatory effects and very low to negligible systemic side effects. They come as sprays, powders and/or drops. Regular use results in improved nasal airflow and olfactory function, and reduced rhinorrhea. The reduction in

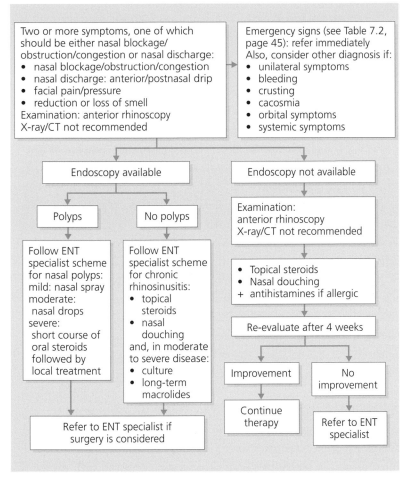

Figure 9.4 A management plan for chronic rhinosinusitis, with or without nasal polyps, in primary care. Adapted from European Position Paper on Rhinosinusitis and Nasal Polyps (EP3OS). *Rhinol Suppl* 2007;20:1–139, with permission (www.rhinologyjournal.com/EPOS2007.pdf).

mucosal swelling and mucus production suggests improved aeration of the mucosa, enabling the sinuses to drain again.

Intranasal steroids are most effective when mucosal contact is optimized. This can be achieved by rinsing the nose some time before spraying and, if obstruction is prominent, opening the nasal cavity with a local decongestant in the first 1–2 weeks of treatment.

The long-term use of nasal corticosteroids does not cause atrophy of mucosa – by contrast with application on skin – and so the prolonged use of intranasal corticosteroids is safe. In addition, there is no contraindication for intranasal corticosteroids during viral infection or exacerbation of chronic sinusitis.

Steroid sprays have the drawback that they only reach the anterior parts of the nose and turbinates, some distance from the site of the problems, namely the middle meatus and ostiomeatal complex. When nasal polyps are present, medication will only reach the foremost bodies of the polyps, not the stalks.

Nasal steroid drops are now available in separate units (nasules) that can be administered in an upside-down position, delivering medication in the middle meatus. These have proven to be effective for nasal polyps, reducing size and symptoms.

If nasal polyps are abundant and nasal airflow is severely impaired, a course of systemic steroids may be needed to open the nose to local treatment. However, in otherwise healthy people, long-term systemic steroid treatment is considered inappropriate. Prednisone or prednisolone, 0.5 mg/kg daily for 1–2 weeks, plus local corticosteroid treatment provide fast subjective relief (within a few days).

Antibiotics. Short-term (< 14 days) antibiotics are often given to people with chronic sinusitis. They give temporary relief, but symptoms often recur after some time. Mucopurulent discharge is often present in individuals with chronic rhinosinusitis. If this is the only symptom, antibiotics are not indicated. Bacteria are usually normal airway pathogens and culture is usually unnecessary and of no additional value because positive cultures are found in approximately 80% of control subjects. Antibiotics should be given if exacerbation occurs and is accompanied by fever, mucosal swelling and increased discharge.

The most frequently encountered bacteria in acute rhinosinusitis are *Streptococcus pneumoniae*, *Haemophilus influenzae* and *Moraxella catarrhalis*. When rhinosinusitis is present for a longer period of time and is more severe, coagulase-negative microorganisms are found: *Staphylococcus aureus*, *Pseudomonas aeruginosa* and Gram-negative agents such as *Enterobacter sp.* Antibiotics that cover these bacteria are:

- amoxicillin/clavulanate, 500/125 mg, three times daily (moderate bone penetration)
- ciprofloxacin, 750 mg, twice daily (high penetration in bone and nasal secretions)
- clarithromycin, 250 mg, twice daily (moderate bone penetration)
- trimethoprim/sulfamethoxazole, 160/800 mg, twice daily (poor bone penetration).

In chronic sinusitis, underlying osteitis is assumed to be present. Bone penetration therefore needs to be taken into consideration as well as mucosal penetration when selecting antibiotics.

If individuals do not respond to these regimens, culture is advised to identify resistant bacteria, and treatment can then target these organisms. Often, people will already have been treated unsuccessfully with courses of antibiotics – the course may not have been long enough or the spectrum may have been too narrow. It is generally accepted that, for chronic rhinosinusitis, 14 days should be the minimum duration of treatment, but refractory rhinosinusitis may require 4–12 weeks' therapy. Controlled trials comparing treatment duration are not available, but given the fact that paranasal sinus bone is involved in chronic rhinosinusitis, it can be reasoned that long-term treatment is needed.

Long-term macrolide therapy. Several studies have described macrolide therapy as having an anti-inflammatory effect in addition to its antibiotic activity. The mechanism is not known, but downregulation of pro-inflammatory cytokines (interleukins IL-6 and IL-8) and inflammatory cells (macrophages and eosinophils) has been observed after treatment with clarithromycin. Treatment with a macrolide for 3 months has been shown to be as effective as surgery.

Anti-allergic measures. Where chronic rhinosinusitis is associated with allergy, the individual should avoid the allergen (see page 63). Additional treatment with local corticosteroid spray and possibly antihistamines should be considered.

If ASA/NSAID hypersensitivity is present, avoidance of all cyclooxygenase-1 (COX-1) inhibitors is mandatory. Some ASA-sensitive individuals report improvement on dietary restriction of additives, preservatives and high-salicylate foods such as herbs, spices and dried fruit, but there is no firm evidence for this.

Local decongestants constrict blood vessels in nasal mucosa, thereby decreasing mucosal thickness and improving nasal airflow. Aeration of the sinuses may also be improved. In addition, local decongestants have antioxidant properties that may have a positive effect on inflammation. On the other hand, it should be stressed and explained to people that local decongestants should not be used for more than 1 week as there is a possibility of a rebound effect.

Antral washouts. The lavage of the maxillary sinus using antral washouts does not result in benefits above those achieved with antibiotics and topical corticosteroids. Nowadays, antral washouts in chronic rhinosinusitis are mainly used for diagnostic purposes.

Antifungal therapy. Fungi have been suggested as having a role in the pathophysiology of all chronic rhinosinusitis. However, several double-blind placebo-controlled trials have shown no effect of antifungal treatment on symptoms and signs of chronic rhinosinusitis with or without nasal polyps.

A subset of individuals suffer from allergic fungal sinusitis (AFS; see Table 9.1, page 90), with positive skin-prick tests to fungi such as *Aspergillus*. AFS is more common in hot and humid climates and it may be associated with allergic bronchopulmonary aspergillosis. Surgery is needed to remove the small quantity of trapped fungus that is stimulating the massive inflammatory response. Following surgery, individuals should continue with douching and topical corticosteroid.

Surgery. If, after optimal medical treatment, symptoms persist, CT imaging should be undertaken. If the CT scan shows opacification of the sinuses (Figure 9.5), indicating mucosal swelling, mucus retention and/or nasal polyps, surgery may be required.

The ostiomeatal complex – the site of drainage and ventilation of most of the paranasal sinuses – is a complex structure and can easily be

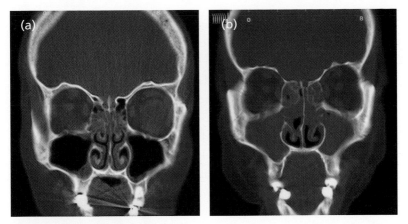

Figure 9.5 CT images of nasal polyposis: (a) early and (b) advanced. Note opacification of sinuses in (b).

obstructed by mucosal swelling (see Figure 9.1). In recent years, it has become apparent that surgery should be functional, only widening the natural drainage openings of the sinuses and preserving as much as possible of the ciliated epithelium that is needed to transport mucus from the sinuses: the functional endoscopic sinus surgery (FESS) technique. This technique emphasizes the natural clearance capacity of the sinuses, making fenestration of the inferior meatus generally unnecessary (except in impaired ciliary function and severe mucus retention).

Key points – rhinosinusitis and nasal polyps

- Viral rhinosinusitis rarely becomes secondarily bacterial.
- Evidence of viral infection can be seen on computed tomography (CT) images taken up to 6 weeks later.
- Acute rhinosinusitis is usually self-limiting.
- Local corticosteroids are first-line treatment for chronic rhinosinusitis.
- Refractory rhinosinusitis may require 4–12 weeks of antibiotic treatment.
- If symptoms persist or are severe, CT imaging should be undertaken and functional surgery may be required.

In the case of nasal polyposis, surgical treatment is generally more aggressive, removing diseased and polypoid mucosa, with the intention of allowing more functional mucosa to return. However, recurrence is often observed in polyposis, particularly in ASA-intolerant individuals, and surgery often needs to be repeated. Because of this, medical treatment with the least bioavailable corticosteroids (fluticasone or mometasone) should be continued after nasal sinus surgery. Usually nasal polyps are removed during endoscopic sinus surgery but they can also be removed in the outpatient clinic with a snare (Figure 9.6).

(a)
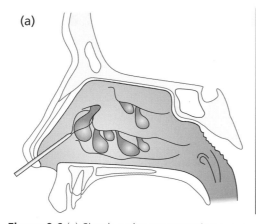

(b)
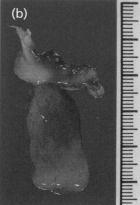

Figure 9.6 (a) Simple polypectomy using a snare. (b) A nasal polyp after removal.

Key references

Bendouah Z, Barbeau J, Hamad WA, Desrosiers M. Biofilm formation by *Staphylococcus aureus* and *Pseudomonas aeruginosa* is associated with an unfavorable evolution after surgery for chronic sinusitis and nasal polyposis. *Otolaryngol Head Neck Surg* 2006;134:991–6.

Fokkens W. Evidence based diagnosis and treatment of rhinosinusitis and nasal polyps. *Rhinology* 2005;43:1.

Fokkens W, Lund V, Mullol J et al. European Position Paper on Rhinosinusitis and Nasal Polyps 2007. *Rhinology* 2007;suppl 20:1–139. www.rhinologyjournal.com/EPOS2007.pdf

Gevaert P, Lang-Loidolt D, Lackner A et al. Nasal IL-5 levels determine the response to anti-IL-5 treatment in patients with nasal polyps. *J Allergy Clin Immunol* 2006;118:1133–41.

Harvey R, Hannan SA, Badia L, Scadding G. Nasal saline irrigations for the symptoms of chronic rhinosinusitis. *Cochrane Database Syst Rev* 2007, issue 3. CD 006394. www.thecochranelibrary.com

Meltzer EO, Hamilos DL, Hadley JA et al. Rhinosinusitis: developing guidance for clinical trials. *J Allergy Clin Immunol* 2006;118(5 suppl): S17–61.

Meltzer EO, Hamilos DL, Hadley JA et al. Rhinosinusitis: establishing definitions for clinical research and patient care. *Otolaryngol Head Neck Surg* 2004;131(6 suppl):S1–62.

Comorbidities and complications of allergic rhinitis

Asthma

Ever since the late 19th century, a relationship has been suspected between upper airway disease and the subsequent development or aggravation of asthma symptoms. To date, the concept of 'one airway, one disease' is generally accepted.

This is supported by common epidemiological, pathological and physiological characteristics. Several studies have demonstrated that both allergic and non-allergic rhinitis are associated with asthma. The underlying mechanism(s) linking these diseases is not fully understood. Possibilities include:

- the loss of the air purification and warming mechanisms of the nose when mouth breathing supervenes
- postnasal dripping of inflammatory mediators during deep sleep
- release of cytokines and mediators from the nasal mucosa to the circulation
- 'homing' of inflammatory cells from the bone marrow to both the upper and lower airways (systemic link)
- naso-sino-bronchial reflex
- abnormalities of upper airway nitric oxide.

Epidemiological evidence suggests that asthma and rhinitis frequently occur as comorbid conditions in the same people, with about 80–90% of people with asthma having rhinitis symptoms and about 20–50% of people with allergic rhinitis having clinical asthma. Furthermore, rhinitis often precedes the onset of clinical asthma and independently increases the risk for developing asthma by up to threefold. It has been proposed that the prevention or early treatment of allergic rhinitis may help to prevent asthma or reduce the severity of bronchial symptoms. Therefore, when considering a diagnosis of rhinitis or asthma, an evaluation of both lower and upper airways should be made.

According to the ARIA (Allergic Rhinitis and its Impact on Asthma) guidelines, people with persistent allergic rhinitis should be evaluated for asthma by history, chest examination and, if possible and when necessary, the assessment of airflow obstruction before and after bronchodilation (see Appendix I). People with asthma should be appropriately evaluated (history and physical examination) for rhinitis. Ideally, a combined strategy should be used to treat the upper and lower airway disease.

Rhinoconjunctivitis

Ocular symptoms occur in a significant proportion of people with rhinitis. From surveys of a large number of people with 'allergic rhinoconjunctivitis', the prevalence of the association between rhinitis and 'conjunctivitis' appears to be different depending on the type of allergy. Allergic conjunctivitis is more common with outdoor allergens than with indoor ones. In some studies of pollen allergy, conjunctivitis is present in over 75% of people suffering from rhinitis.

Allergic eye diseases represent a heterogeneous entity, including different forms of conjunctivitis with different signs, symptoms, pathophysiology, degree of severity and response to treatment. Severe forms, such as vernal conjunctivitis, tend to occur in young boys and require ophthalmic expertise as topical corticosteroids may be required and close monitoring of the eyes with a slit lamp is necessary.

Treatment. Avoidance measures include wearing wrap-around sunglasses and topical douching with sterile saline drops.

The first treatment choice in rhinoconjunctivitis is topical or oral antihistamines. Topical antihistamines provide faster and more effective relief than systemic antihistamines. Topical vasoconstrictors provide rapid relief, particularly for redness; however, the relief is often short-lived, and overuse of vasoconstrictors may lead to rebound hyperemia and irritation. Another class of topical agents, mast cell stabilizers (sodium cromoglicate [cromolyn sodium], nedocromil and lodoxamide), may be considered; however, they generally have a much slower onset of action and are best used prophylactically, starting pre-seasonally and using regularly. Lastly, topical corticosteroids may be considered for severe seasonal ocular allergy symptoms under expert supervision, though long-term use should be avoided because of risks of ocular adverse effects, including herpetic keratitis, glaucoma and cataract formation.

All ocular preparations contain preservatives such as benzalkonium chloride to which some people are hypersensitive. Use with soft contact lenses is contraindicated; hard lenses must be removed before use and re-inserted after 10 minutes.

Adenoid hypertrophy

The adenoid is the peripheral lymphoid organ located in the nasopharynx. It forms part of Waldeyer's ring and contributes to the development of immunity against inhaled microorganisms in early life. Many triggers, including microbial stimuli such as molds or external irritants like cigarette smoke, have been related to the enlargement of adenoid tissue and hence to the development of symptoms. Symptoms related to adenoid hypertrophy range from nasal obstruction, rhinolalia, hyponasal voice, open-mouth breathing and snoring, to sleep apnea. Signs include the so-called 'adenoid facies' (see Figure 7.1, page 46).

In children, both allergic rhinitis and adenoid hypertrophy may give rise to similar symptoms, and therefore need to be differentiated at the time of the consultation. This is not always easy, as there is no good method of assessment other than nasendoscopy: acoustic rhinometry is unreliable far back in the nose and lateral X-rays can be influenced by swallowing. A trial of rhinitis treatment using topical corticosteroids is sensible under these circumstances as these pass postnasally and can reduce adenoid tissue. Children with marked sleep apnea and daytime somnolence need referral to ear, nose and throat (ENT) services.

Although the role of allergy is unclear in adenoid hypertrophy, allergy should be investigated in children with symptomatic adenoid hypertrophy.

Nasal steroids are capable of reducing adenoid-related symptoms with no differences in response between atopic and non-atopic children. In studies, the effects of nasal steroids on symptoms of allergic inflammation in the nose and adenoid cannot be dissociated from their anti-inflammatory effects on the adenoid itself. Properly conducted clinical trials on antihistamines in allergic children with allergic rhinitis and adenoid hypertrophy are lacking.

Tubal dysfunction

The eustachian tube exerts a major function in middle-ear homeostasis via its role in the ventilation and protection of the middle ear and mucociliary clearance. People with allergic rhinitis have a higher risk of eustachian tube dysfunction assessed by tympanometry than non-allergic people, particularly during childhood.

Otitis media with effusion

OME is an inflammatory disease of the middle-ear mucosa and it remains a significant problem in children. It is estimated that more than 80% of all children have at least one episode of otitis media by the age of 3 years and that 40% will have three or more episodes.

Immunoglobulin E sensitization and respiratory allergy symptoms are independent risk factors for the development of OME. The middle-ear fluid of atopic people with OME contains more eosinophils and cells positive for interleukins IL-4 and IL-5 mRNA than that of non-atopic individuals with OME, suggestive of a role of allergic inflammation in OME.

It remains difficult to interpret epidemiological data as we cannot estimate to what extent the enhanced prevalence of allergy in people with OME, reported by some authors, represents a true finding or rather reflects a referral bias. A recent epidemiological questionnaire study in first-year school children in the Slough and Windsor area in the UK notes a very strong association between symptoms of OME and those of rhinitis. It is proposed that children with recurrent OME should be asked about nasal symptoms, examined for rhinitis and tested for allergy. A few studies have now shown that treatment of noses with topical corticosteroids aids resolution of OME, probably because eustachian tube function and middle-ear ventilation are improved.

Pharyngitis/laryngitis

People who breathe chronically through their mouths have dry mouths and tend to suffer from sore throats. Postnasal secretions dripping down into the pharynx and on to the larynx can also cause irritation, resulting in coughing and hawking. This, in turn, results in further local irritation of the mucous membranes, and thus a vicious circle is created. Such symptoms are very difficult to resolve completely; postnasal passage of mucus is a normal phenomenon and once it has been noticed, the perception of it tends to persist even if the volume and stickiness of the secretions have been reduced by treatment of the rhinosinusitis.

Key points – comorbidities and complications of allergic rhinitis

- Rhinitis, both allergic and non-allergic, is associated with effects on surrounding structures: eyes, sinuses, throat, ears and lower airways.
- Rhinitis may appear first and be causative.
- Adequate treatment of rhinitis can have ameliorating effects.
- Individuals with otitis media with effusion, pharyngitis, laryngitis, sleep problems and/or asthma or chronic cough need thorough investigation for concomitant rhinitis plus adequate treatment if present.

Key references

Bousquet J, Van Cauwenberge P, Khaltaev N. Allergic rhinitis and its impact on asthma. *J Allergy Clin Immunol* 2001;108(5 suppl):S147–334. www.whiar.org/pocketguide/one.html

Ciprandi G, Cirillo I. The lower airway pathology of rhinitis. *J Allergy Clin Immunol* 2006; 118:1105–9.

Fokkens W, Lund V, Mullol J et al. European Position Paper on Rhinosinusitis and Nasal Polyps 2007. *Rhinology* 2007;suppl 20: 1–139.

Hellings PW, Fokkens WJ. Allergic rhinitis and its impact on otorhinolaryngology. *Allergy* 2006;61:656–64.

Hens G, Hellings PW. The nose: gatekeeper and trigger of bronchial disease. *Rhinology* 2006;44:179–87.

Jeffery PK, Haahtela T. Allergic rhinitis and asthma: inflammation in a one-airway condition. *BMC Pulm Med* 2006;30;6(suppl 1):S5.

Umapathy D, Alles R, Scadding GK. A community-based questionnaire study on the association between symptoms suggestive of otitis media with effusion, rhinitis and asthma in primary school children. *Int J Pediatr Otorhinolaryngol* 2007;71:705–12.

Xu Z, Cheuk DK, Lee SL. Clinical evaluation in predicting childhood obstructive sleep apnea. *Chest* 2006; 130:1765–71.

Allergic rhinitis

One in three teenagers has allergic disease according to a recent UK survey that used the International Study of Asthma and Allergies in Childhood (ISAAC) questionnaire. Similar surveys show rhinitis to be increasingly prevalent in many areas worldwide. Climate change is likely to alter pollen patterns and timings so allergens such as *Parietaria*, olive and ragweed may become important in the UK.

Prevention. Until the factors causing the increase in allergic diseases are fully discovered, prevention will remain problematic. The dietary use of bacteria and their products early in life (probiotics) has reduced the incidence of atopic eczema but not that of subsequent asthma or rhinitis. Further work is in progress.

Studies looking at the effects of reducing exposure to traffic pollution and cigarette smoke and of dietary supplementation with antioxidants are ongoing.

Treatment. Many people are unwilling to use long-term topical nasal steroids. If sublingual immunotherapy has long-term benefits (prevention of new sensitization and progression to asthma), such as those seen with injection immunotherapy, then it is likely to be widely used as therapy in combination with secondary prevention.

There is a possibility that initial exposure to allergen via the mouth and gut, rather than into the airways, might result in tolerance, so investigation of sublingual allergens as primary prevention is likely. However, the costs and availability of large quantities of allergen could limit these approaches.

Other vaccines are under development, including those using allergen combined with fragments from bacterial DNA (CpG motifs not found in man) – these look promising.

The possibility of developing autoimmunity to DNA needs to be monitored.

Peptide fragments of allergen alter T cell responses without causing mast cell degranulation. Late adverse reactions have occurred, however.

Monoclonal antibodies to cytokines and other molecules involved in the allergic reaction (anti-immunoglobulin E [IgE], anti-interleukin-5 [IL-5], anti-IL-4, anti-eotaxin) have been investigated. Of these, only anti-IgE has reached the clinic and its place there is limited by cost. An approach using small molecule inhibitors is likely to prove cheaper.

A combined approach to treating both upper and lower airway disease is being encouraged. Ideally, an oral therapy will be found that controls both with minimal side effects.

Non-allergic rhinitis

Elucidation of the mechanisms underlying non-allergic rhinitis is needed before logical therapy can be provided. Eosinophilic forms, particularly in acetylsalicylic acid-sensitive individuals, may respond to antileukotrienes. Neurological forms will require specific treatment, possibly directed at higher nervous levels to prevent excessive transmitter release or sensitivity.

Chronic rhinosinusitis and nasal polyps

International, multicenter clinical trials should be used in well-characterized individuals using multiple outcome measures, including symptoms, quality of life and effects on both upper and lower airways, to further determine the effect of different forms of treatment.

Endoscopic sinus surgery is less likely to be used as medical therapy improves. The role of bacteria in stimulating nasal polyps and the possible biofilm causation of chronic rhinosinusitis may lead to targeted topical therapy.

Key references

Bousquet J, van Cauwenberge P, Aït Khaled N et al. Pharmacologic and anti-IgE treatment of allergic rhinitis: ARIA update (in collaboration with GA2LEN). *Allergy* 2006;61:1086–96.

Didier A. Future developments in sublingual immunotherapy. *Allergy* 2006;61(suppl 81):29–31.

Emberlin J. The effects of patterns in climate and pollen abundance on allergy. *Allergy* 1994;49(suppl 18): 15–20.

Meltzer EO, Hamilos DL, Hadley JA et al. Rhinosinusitis: developing guidance for clinical trials. *J Allergy Clin Immunol* 2006;118(5 suppl): S17–61.

Owen CE. Immunoglobulin E: role in asthma and allergic disease: lessons from the clinic. *Pharmacol Ther* 2007;113:121–33.

Appendix I

Allergic Rhinitis and its Impact on Asthma (ARIA) guidelines

- First truly global guidelines
- Redefine rhinitis
- Consider comorbidities
- Evidence-based approach to management
- Specific recommendations cover:
  - allergic rhinitis classified as a major chronic respiratory disease because of its:
    - prevalence
    - impact on quality of life
    - impact on work/school performance and productivity
    - economic burden
    - links with asthma
    - association with sinusitis and other comorbidities such as conjunctivitis
  - allergic rhinitis considered as a risk factor for asthma
  - a new subdivision of allergic rhinitis: intermittent; persistent
  - allergic rhinitis classified as 'mild' or 'moderate/severe'
  - a stepwise therapeutic approach
  - treatment should combine: allergen avoidance (when possible), pharmacotherapy, immunotherapy
  - optimization of environmental and social factors
  - evaluation of patients with persistent allergic rhinitis for asthma by history, by chest examination and, if possible, by the assessment of airflow obstruction before and after a bronchodilator
  - evaluation of patients with asthma for rhinitis
  - a combined strategy for treating coexistent upper and lower airway diseases
  - a specific strategy for developing countries depending on available treatments and interventions and their cost

Source: Bousquet J, Van Cauwenberge P, Khaltaev N. Allergic rhinitis and its impact on asthma. *J Allergy Clin Immunol* 2001;108(5 suppl):S147–334 (www.whiar.org/pocketguide/one.html).

Appendix II

Frequently asked questions

Why bother treating a runny nose? My drugs budget is tight. Can't rhinitis sufferers just buy tissues and get on with it?

Rhinitis is more than just a runny nose for many sufferers. The symptoms of nasal blocking, itching and sneezing together with rhinorrhea can disrupt their lives – the effect on quality of life is equivalent to that of chronic back pain or angina, and it has an impact greater than mild to moderate asthma. There are also secondary effects including poor quality of sleep, which interferes with workplace and school attendance and performance.

In addition, rhinitis is likely to progress to asthma, to sinusitis and, in children, is associated with otitis media with effusion.

There is evidence that treatment of rhinitis improves quality of life, work and school attendance and can reduce asthma exacerbations and the need for grommets, so it is likely to be cost-effective.

How do I start?

The first thing is to decide if your patient really has rhinitis, how often, how severely, and then, if possible, what kind of rhinitis it is.

Take a history, asking about which symptoms are present: running, blocking, itching and sneezing. Find out which symptoms bother the patient most and whether the symptoms interfere with their life. Ask about when they occur and how long they last. Check for comorbidities such as asthma, sinusitis, and ear, throat and sleep problems.

Then determine whether the problem is mild or moderate to severe using the ARIA guidelines (see Figure 4.1 and Appendix I) and whether it is intermittent or persistent. Treatment is based on this classification (see Figure 8.3, page 69).

Take a look at, and up, the nose – an allergic crease may be visible – large pale turbinates and clear secretions also suggest allergic rhinitis.

The ARIA guidelines mention allergen avoidance – how can I diagnose allergies in primary care?

Allergy diagnosis rests mainly on a detailed history – primary care practitioners are ideally placed as they probably know a lot about the circumstances of their patients' lives – housing, pets, occupation. Ask when symptoms occur in relation to possible allergen exposure – is there an improvement away from home, are symptoms work-related or seasonal? A clear history of rhinitis starting in mid May and ending in late July (in the UK) is strongly suggestive of grass pollen allergy, in which case specific tests for allergy antibodies are only needed if immunotherapy is contemplated. When the history is less clear, specific tests (skin-prick or blood tests for specific immunoglobulin E [IgE]), are helpful.

Skin-prick tests are too dangerous for use in my surgery, aren't they?

Skin-prick tests were no more dangerous than taking blood in a survey of 10 000 individuals. Provided only inhalant allergens are used there is no reason why a trained primary care provider should not undertake skin-prick tests. Injectable epinephrine should be immediately available, together with resuscitation equipment, but these are very unlikely to be needed.

Skin-prick tests need to be properly performed and interpreted, so some training is necessary – this is now available in the UK (see www.bsaci.org).

Allergen avoidance doesn't work though, does it?

Properly performed, allergen avoidance works extremely well. For example, hay fever sufferers are asymptomatic outside the grass pollen season, and latex allergen avoidance by the use of non-powdered gloves or ones made of nitrile has reduced symptoms in healthcare workers. High-quality studies using one modality of house dust mite avoidance have not shown efficacy in rhinitis or asthma, but a recent, small, open study in children using multiple modalities for house dust mites plus pet removal and superheated steam cleaning showed dramatic improvements in rhinitis and asthma. It is likely that a concerted approach to all major allergens is needed and that this may be most effective early in the disease (i.e. in rhinitis sufferers before asthma develops, and possibly in children more than adults).

What if the skin-prick tests are negative? What do I do then?

Negative skin-prick tests can occur if the person has been taking antihistamines or has had topical corticosteroids on the skin surface used for testing. Other explanations are that the correct allergen was not tested for – recheck the history for other possible causes – or that the allergic sensitization is localized in the nose (a phenomenon recognized in childhood and in some adults) or that a non-allergic form of rhinitis is involved. This could arise from infection – children have many colds per year – or there may be another cause of rhinitis.

In primary care, a trial of rhinitis treatment with topical nasal corticosteroids is sensible as some forms of non-allergic rhinitis respond to this. Failure should lead to specialist referral.

Who else should I refer to a specialist? And which specialist?

Ear, nose and throat (ENT) referral is needed for those people with unilateral symptoms or signs, bloodstained mucus, new polyps and very severe or refractive symptoms.

Allergy referral may help for those who have an allergic rhinitis unresponsive to treatment or a suspected but undiagnosed allergy.

My patient is well controlled on topical nasal corticosteroids – but I can't keep prescribing them, can I?

It is interesting how primary care providers are willing to continue prescribing inhaled corticosteroids for asthma but unwilling to do the same with intranasal ones for rhinitis. The inflammatory pathway is the same in both disorders. Indeed, there is now a one-airway approach suggesting that the upper airway is always involved to some extent in asthma and often requires treatment. Worries about long-term safety are largely unfounded if the least bioavailable molecules are used.

Corticosteroids do not damage the nasal lining, though they may cause minor epistaxis, particularly if wrongly used so that septal deposition of the dose occurs all in one place. Systemic absorption occurs to a small extent through the nasal mucosa and also through the gut as most of the dose is swallowed. This varies according to the molecules used – it is high with betamethasone and dexamethasone and less than 1% with the newer therapies fluticasone and mometasone.

111

Children's growth should be monitored as they may be receiving corticosteroids at three sites for asthma, eczema and rhinitis. Adults with glaucoma should receive an alternative form of treatment. A study of 20 000 intranasal steroid users suggested no increased risk of cataracts.

Appendix III

Case studies
Case study 1 – seasonal allergic rhinitis

Clare was 14 when she first noticed that she had a problem with 'summer colds'. The symptoms were not so bad and she did not seek treatment.

She was fine all winter. Next summer she was revising hard for her examinations when the colds began again. This year they were worse and she had a continually runny nose, sneezed and had itchy, red eyes. Being a teenager, she did not seek adult advice but asked her friends, who told her she probably had hay fever and that she should buy some treatment from the local pharmacist. This she did; the pharmacist suggested an oral antihistamine. Clare asked for the cheapest one and was given chlorphenamine.

She started taking one tablet at night as directed. Unfortunately, though her nasal and eye symptoms improved she found it hard to get up in the morning and was drowsy during the day. It was a real effort to do any revision.

Her results were poorer than expected and provoked an enquiry from her teachers. Luckily, one of them knew about the psychomotor retardation and sedation side effects of the first-generation antihistamines, having experienced them herself. She suggested that Clare should see her primary care provider about hay fever so that the problem could be solved before Clare's important GCSE examinations the following summer.

Clare's doctor took a history and found that Clare's symptoms began in May and continued until the end of July – the typical grass pollen season in the UK. She noted that Clare's eyes and nose were affected and that her worst symptoms were running and itching. As the symptoms occurred for more than 4 days at a time for more than 4 weeks, Clare had persistent rhinitis, and because her schooling was affected it was moderate to severe. The ARIA guidelines suggested topical corticosteroids as first-line therapy with an additional non-sedating antihistamine if needed. They also advised starting treatment early (i.e. 2 weeks before symptoms usually started) and using it regularly, rather than 'as needed'.

The following year, Clare began using a topical nasal corticosteroid plus a non-sedating antihistamine in early May. She used both every day until the end of July and hardly noticed any hay fever symptoms. She did very well in her examinations.

Learning points

- Seasonal allergic rhinitis is not necessarily intermittent and is often not mild.
- It frequently requires more than one medication to achieve reasonable symptom control.
- Starting therapy early with intranasal corticosteroids delays the onset of symptoms and reduces their severity.
- Regular treatment is more effective than symptom-directed therapy.
- Sedating antihistamines should not be used to treat rhinitis. A teenager using these has a 70% chance of dropping a grade in one subject at GCSE compared with their mock examination grade.

Additional message

For people with hay fever that does not respond to the above measures, grass pollen-specific immunotherapy should be considered. Subcutaneous immunotherapy is only available in a few specialist centers in the UK, but sublingual immunotherapy with grass pollen tablets is now licensed for use. This must be started under supervision, but after the first dose the tablets are taken daily at home, starting 8 weeks pre-seasonally and continuing throughout the season. There is a reduction in symptoms of about one-third in the first year of use, with a similar reduction in the need for medication.

Continuous therapy for 3 years is under investigation at present to see if it has the same effects as 3 years of subcutaneous immunotherapy (i.e. at least 4 further years of remission and a reduction in the progression to further allergic sensitization and asthma).

Case study 2 – multiple food allergies

David was sent to the allergy clinic with a note from his concerned doctor: "Please see this man urgently as he has suddenly developed reactions to nuts and other foods and these are increasing."

David gave a history of being able to eat all nuts without problems until the previous spring, when he found that hazelnuts and almonds irritated his mouth and tongue. He avoided them until Christmas when he ate a chocolate-covered roast almond without problems. Next spring he developed a similar problem with some fruits, most notably apples. Raw apples made his lips and mouth itchy and also irritated his throat. He had no difficulty with apple pie. Cherries and nectarines, carrots and celery had recently produced similar effects. He had no difficulty in breathing and no systemic symptoms.

On direct questioning he admitted to having had rhinitis each spring for the past 8 years, but no other allergies. Physical examination including mouth and throat was normal.

Skin-prick testing was positive to birch tree pollen, hazel pollen, hazelnut and almond. Commercial extracts of apple and carrot were negative; nectarine and cherry were unavailable.

Prick-to-prick testing (inserting a needle directly into the fruit and then into the patient's skin) using the raw fruits gave positive results.

Learning points

- David has the oral allergy syndrome in which sensitization to pollen causes cross-reactivity to similar molecules found in nuts, fruit and vegetables.
- It is a localized reaction and is rarely very severe, though in some individuals throat swelling can occur. If severe, epinephrine should be prescribed – either as a spray or injection.
- The clue is that once cooked, the fruit is tolerated as the relevant allergens are heat-labile. This also accounts for the unreliability of commercial extracts for skin-prick testing in these individuals and the value of testing with the fresh raw food.
- The symptoms tend to worsen during the relevant pollen season as IgE levels increase. Regular antihistamines may help.

Case study 3 – recurrent otitis media with effusion

Sam, aged 6, attended the pediatric ENT/allergy clinic with his mother, who complained that Sam's hearing had declined again. This had happened over a year before after a cold, and when it had lasted 3 months he'd had grommets inserted. These restored his hearing to normal, then fell out after about 6 months, but Sam had been able to hear reasonably well until he went back to school in September and caught a cold within 2 weeks. Now his teacher was complaining that Sam was not paying attention in class and was not making good progress. His mother wanted "something doing – but not more grommets".

On going into the history, Sam also had a blocked and runny nose which he rubbed frequently. He snored at night and sneezed in the mornings. These symptoms began when the family moved house 2 years before to an old and dusty house where several cats had lived with an elderly lady.

As a baby Sam had had mild transient eczema. His father had hay fever. Examination revealed a boy who was a chronic mouth breather with an allergic crease across his nose. His inferior turbinates were pale, wet and swollen. There were mucopurulent secretions in both sides of his nose. Both eardrums were dull. His chest was clear and he had a normal peak flow reading. Tympanograms were flat bilaterally; hearing levels for speech averaged 25 dB on both sides.

A diagnosis of rhinitis and otitis media with effusion was made. Sam and his mother agreed to skin-prick testing. This showed a positive reaction to cat and house dust mite.

The doctor explained that the two conditions might be linked as natural ventilation and drainage of the middle ear takes place via the eustachian tube which leads into the back of the nose. The two organs have the same lining, which was probably inflamed because of the allergies, thus decreasing normal eustachian tube function and leaving the middle ear more susceptible to fluid accumulation.

He proposed a 3-month rhinitis treatment period while waiting to see if the effusion disappeared; if it did not, grommets could be considered at that stage.

Sam's mother initially agreed and the doctor explained that the rhinitis treatment involved allergen avoidance measures at home: removal of the ancient carpet and steam cleaning of Sam's bedroom followed by allergen-proof bed covers. Weekly changing of bed linen with hot washing, vacuuming and damp dusting was to be instituted. His mother was happy to undertake this but she did not initially want Sam to have the steroid spray once daily as the doctor prescribed. Her fears were allayed when he told her that the spray was only absorbed into Sam in minute quantities and that it acted directly on the lining of the nose, which it would not damage.

Sam was shown how to use the spray and was encouraged to have a go with the dummy spray provided. He agreed to give one puff in each nostril once a day, immediately before cleaning his teeth. Both he and his mum were warned that the effects of treatment would not appear for a couple of weeks.

A 3-month follow-up was arranged.

When reviewed, both Sam and his mother were very happy. She had undertaken good allergen avoidance measures and Sam had taken the spray and continued, as asked, with a second one from his family practitioner. Within 2 weeks his nose had cleared and he had begun to sleep better without snoring. He was easier to wake up in the morning. His hearing had returned to normal and he was doing well at school.

Examination showed a good nasal airway and no more nose rubbing. Hearing tests were normal.

Learning points
- Nasal inflammation often extends to involve adjacent structures such as sinuses, ears, throat and lower respiratory tract, which are all lined with pseudostratified respiratory epithelium.
- Inflammation and infection can summate – viral colds precipitate exacerbations of sinusitis, polyps, asthma and otitis media more often in allergic individuals, particularly if they are exposed to their allergens.

Case study 4 – child with a runny nose

Mehmet, aged 5, was brought to the ENT clinic by his mother, who spoke little English. The history appeared to be of a continual, unrelenting mucopurulent nasal discharge, present for a long time, accompanied by nasal obstruction and snoring. He also had a long-standing hearing problem and a wet cough, for which his doctor had prescribed two inhalers: one containing corticosteroid, the other salbutamol. These were rarely used as they did not improve his symptoms. He was otherwise well and had no past history of eczema. There was no family history of atopy, but a cousin had similar symptoms.

Examination revealed a slight boy on the 10th centile for weight and height who was mouth breathing. There was a thick white discharge present in both nostrils, with swollen pale inferior turbinates. Both eardrums were dull. His chest was indrawn around the lower intercostal area and there were one or two wheezes audible on auscultation. Hearing tests showed bilateral flat tympanograms with hearing levels over the speech range at 40 dB.

The ENT surgeon diagnosed otitis media with effusion and probable adenoid hypertrophy and listed him for grommet insertion and examination of the postnasal space under anesthesia.

When Mehmet was admitted a few weeks later, the anesthetist was not satisfied with the chest examination and organized a preoperative chest X-ray. This revealed dextrocardia, which led to a diagnosis of primary ciliary dyskinesia (PCD). The operation was cancelled because grommet insertion in people with PCD causes chronic ear discharge. Hearing difficulties usually resolve with increasing age and are best managed by hearing aids.

Learning points
- PCD is present in around 1 in 10 000 of the population, but is more common in some ethnic groups. Early diagnosis is vital as lifelong chest physiotherapy is needed to remove secretions and prevent bronchiectasis. The diagnosis should always be considered in children with a history of a wet cough from birth who respond poorly to asthma medications; most also have chronic, unremitting rhinorrhea,

and otitis media with effusion is common. Only 50% of sufferers have dextrocardia, so diagnosis is made on ciliary structure and function studies undertaken at specialized centers, of which there are three in the UK. Recently, the observation that nasal nitric oxide is very low in PCD has been useful in excluding the diagnosis – a level of 250 ppb excludes PCD with 95% sensitivity.

- There is no specific therapy for the nasal discharge, but regular saline douching is helpful in clearing secretions.

Useful resources

UK

Action Against Allergy
PO Box 278
Twickenham TW1 4QQ
Tel: +44 (0)20 8892 2711
AAA@actionagainstallergy.
freeserve.co.uk
www.actionagainstallergy.co.uk

Allergy UK
(British Allergy Foundation)
3 White Oak Square, London Road
Swanley, Kent BR8 7AG
Helpline: +44 (0)1322 619898
info@allergyuk.org
www.allergyuk.org

Asthma UK
Summit House, 70 Wilson Street
London EC2A 2DB
Helpline: 08457 010203
Tel: 08456 038143
info@asthma.org.uk
www.asthma.org.uk

British Society for Allergy & Clinical Immunology
17 Doughty Street
London WC1N 2PL
Tel: +44 (0)20 7404 0278
info@bsaci.org
www.bsaci.org

USA

American Academy of Allergy, Asthma & Immunology
555 East Wells Street, Suite 1100
Milwaukee, WI 53202-3823
Tel: +1 414 272 6071
Helpline: 1 800 822 2762
info@aaaai.org
www.aaaai.org

American Association for Respiratory Care
9425 N. MacArthur Blvd
Suite 100, Irving, TX 75063-4706
Tel: +1 972 243 2272
info@aarc.org
www.aarc.org

American College of Allergy, Asthma & Immunology
85 West Algonquin Road
Suite 550, Arlington Heights
IL 60005
Tel: +1 847 427 1200
mail@acaai.org
www.acaai.org

Respiratory Nursing Society
c/o Casey Norris
708 Gladstone CR
Maryville, TN 37804
CNorris@etch.com
www.respiratorynursingsociety.org

International

Australasian Rhinologic Society
www.ars.org.au

Canadian Society of Allergy & Clinical Immunology
774 Echo Drive
Ottawa, ON, K1S 5N8
Tel: +1 613 730 6272
csaci@rcpsc.edu
www.csaci.medical.org

European Academy of Allergology & Clinical Immunology
Executive Office, PO Box 24140
S-104 51 Stockholm, Sweden
Tel: +46 8 459 66 23
executive.office@eaaci.org
www.eaaci.net

European Respiratory Care Association
11 chemin Beau Site
1004 Lausanne, Switzerland
Tel: +33 607 69 22 85
(President – Philippe Joud)
philippe.joud@eurorespicare.com
www.eurorespicare.com

European Rhinologic Society
www.europeanrhinologicsociety.org

Global Allergy & Asthma European Network
www.ga2len.net

International Primary Care Respiratory Group
www.theipcrg.org

World Allergy Organization
WAO Secretariat
555 East Wells Street
Suite 1100, Milwaukee
WI 53202-3823, USA
Tel: +1 414 276 1791
info@worldallergy.org
www.worldallergy.org

Further reading

ARIA guidelines. Management of Allergic Rhinitis and its Impact on Asthma Initiative pocket guide www.whiar.org/pocketguide/one.html

Fokkens W, Lund V, Mullol J et al. European Position Paper on Rhinosinusitis and Nasal Polyps 2007. *Rhinology* 2007;suppl20: 1–139. www.rhinologyjournal.com /EPOS2007.pdf

Scadding G, Lund VJ. *Investigative Rhinology*. London, New York: Taylor & Francis, 2004.

Index